T0225091

Clinical Cases in Dysphagia

Dysphagia is a complex condition that can have significant social, developmental and psychological effects. Alongside the physiology and pathophysiology of the condition, dysphagia can rob patients of the most basic pleasures, such as eating and drinking, causing ongoing difficulties for individuals in social situations throughout the lifespan.

As an acknowledged component of evidence-based practice, the humble case report encourages clinical reflection and may be the spark that generates new thinking and motivation for future research. *Clinical Cases in Dysphagia* provides an opportunity to gain insight into the unique and varied presentation and management of dysphagia across a range of different conditions. With chapters provided by expert clinicians and based on clinical examples 'from the trenches', the reader may gain insights into their own practice patterns, refine their clinical problem solving and better value the education that is offered to each of us by our patients.

With additional online resources to support the case-based approach, the book emphasizes the importance of multidisciplinary care and reflects everyday clinical practice, making it a must-read for clinicians and students.

Margaret Walshe, PhD, is an Associate Professor and Head of Department of Clinical Speech and Language Studies at Trinity College Dublin. She has over 30 years' clinical experience in swallowing disorders and was instrumental in establishing the first postgraduate courses in dysphagia in the Republic of Ireland. She is a Vice-President of the European Society for Swallowing Disorders. Her research interests are acquired neurological dysphagia, implementation science and evidence-based practice.

Maggie-Lee Huckabee, PhD, worked clinically for 15 years before returning to university for a research degree. She is now a Professor in the Department of Communication Disorders, the University of Canterbury and Director of the Rose Centre for Stroke Recovery and Research at St Georges Medical Centre in Christchurch New Zealand. Her research interests focus on the complexities of behaviourally driven neural adaptation and biomechanical change leading to swallowing recovery.

Clinical Cases in Speech and Language Disorders

Clinical Cases in Speech and Language Disorders is a new series of short books that each focus on a specific speech and language disorder, providing an in-depth look at real or imagined scenarios, and discussing relevant assessment and intervention plans using theory, research findings, and clinical reasoning. The overall aim of these books is to provide much-needed resources using real-life clinical cases to help clinicians and students reflect on clinical decision making involving the assessment and management of patients presenting with various speech and language disorders (SLD).

Titles in the series:

Clinical Cases in Dysphagia
Edited by Margaret Walshe and Maggie-Lee Huckabee

For more information about this series, please visit: https://www.routledge.com/Clinical-Cases-in-Speech-and-Language-Disorders/book-series/CCSLD

Clinical Cases in Dysphagia

Edited by Margaret Walshe and
Maggie-Lee Huckabee

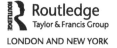
Routledge
Taylor & Francis Group

LONDON AND NEW YORK

First published 2019
by Routledge
2 Park Square, Milton Park, Abingdon, Oxon OX14 4RN

and by Routledge
711 Third Avenue, New York, NY 10017

Routledge is an imprint of the Taylor & Francis Group, an informa business

© 2019 selection and editorial matter, Margaret Walshe and Maggie-Lee Huckabee; individual chapters, the contributors

British Library Cataloguing-in-Publication Data
A catalogue record for this book is available from the British Library

Library of Congress Cataloging-in-Publication Data
A catalog record has been requested for this book

ISBN: 978-1-138-08754-5 (hbk)
ISBN: 978-1-138-08761-3 (pbk)
ISBN: 978-1-315-11036-3 (ebk)

Typeset in Sabon
by Swales & Willis Ltd, Exeter, Devon, UK

Please visit the eResource at www.routledge.com/9781138087613

Dedication and acknowledgement

As researchers who were both initially clinicians, we well recognize that our best teachers for understanding dysphagia and its management are our patients. This book is dedicated to these patients, who challenge our thinking, tolerate our inadequacies and patiently (or not) wait for us to find the answers to alleviate the outcomes of their impairment. It is through their idiosyncrasies that we learn to stretch our thinking and create new management approaches.

Great regard is given to the clinicians who we chose to contribute because they very likely share these beliefs. We thank them for sharing what they have learned through their clinical engagement with those who depend on us for care.

Contents

List of illustrations

Supplementary (Suppl) materials available on the eResource page at www.routledge.com/9781138087613

Tables

Figures

Supplementary material

Contributors

Sasha Adams graduated with a Bachelor degree (first class honours) in speech and language pathology at the University of Canterbury in New Zealand in 2017. She completed an honours project in the area of paediatric dysphagia under the supervision of Professor Maggie-Lee Huckabee. Since then, she has been based in a clinical role in the area of neurorehabilitation for a district health board. She has a particular interest in the area of adult and paediatric dysphagia.

Grainne Brady is the Clinical Lead Speech and Language Therapist at the Royal Marsden NHS Foundation Trust. Since completing her undergraduate degree at Trinity College Dublin in 2008, she has worked at specialist oncology and head and neck cancer centres in Ireland, before moving to the Royal Marsden NHS Foundation Trust in London in 2013. She was awarded her National Institute for Health Research (NIHR)-funded Master's in Research by St George's, University of London in 2016. Grainne's research interests include head and neck cancer, dysphagia in lung cancer and palliative care.

Marion Dolan is a speech and language therapist who has worked for the past 7 years with the Health Services Executive in Ireland, Enable Ireland, Dublin and in a research capacity with Trinity College Dublin. Marion's interest in dementia arose from personal experience of caring for a close relative with dementia. She has completed research on modifying the acute hospital ward environment to facilitate communication for people with dementia and was awarded Trinity College Dublin's Beggs Leask Prize for this research.

Éadaoin Flynn is Senior Speech and Language Therapist at Tallaght University Hospital, Dublin. She has extensive clinical experience in dysphagia assessment and management with a variety of populations presenting with neurological conditions. Her dysphagia research

interests include diet modification as an intervention for oropharyngeal dysphagia in people with dementia, respiratory–swallowing
coordination, videofluoroscopy and radiation practices. She has an
MSc specializing in dysphagia from Trinity College Dublin. She is
also a Cochrane Research Fellow and is involved with the Cochrane
Dementia and Cognitive Improvement Group.

Katrin Frank is a physiotherapist und respiratory therapist. She has
worked in acute care and early neurorehabilitation settings since 1997,
with a focus on tracheotomized patients with and without dysphagia,
ventilator weaning and management of respiratory disorders. Besides
leading and working with an interdisciplinary team of physiotherapists, occupational therapists, and speech and language therapists she
develops and validates respiratory intervention concepts. She enjoys
teaching other clinical teams to improve their interdisciplinary dysphagia management and integrate respiratory treatment approaches
into their dysphagia intervention programmes.

Ulrike Frank worked as a speech–language therapist in early neurorehabilitation from 1997 to 2004 and then shifted her workplace to a
university environment, where she finished her PhD by developing an
interdisciplinary tracheostomy-weaning concept. She enjoys teaching
students to understand physiology and impairments of swallowing
and speaking, and to do their first research steps in the Swallowing
Research Lab that she founded in 2009. Furthermore, she has a great
time with Katrin Frank teaching clinical teams in interdisciplinary
dysphagia treatment workshops.

Kristin Gozdzikowska began clinical work as a speech–language therapist in acute care and inpatient rehabilitation, developing a specific
interest in the assessment and management of dysphagia. She received
her Master's degree at the University of Washington in 2011 and her
Doctoral degree at the University of Canterbury, New Zealand, in
2016. Currently, she is a Post-Doctoral Fellow at the University of
Canterbury Rose Centre for Stroke Recovery and Research and a
speech–language therapist working with patients after moderate-to-
severe brain injury at Laura Fergusson Trust. Her research interests
include best practice in instrumental assessment and rehabilitation of
dysphagia following stroke, contributing to the evidence base from
which clinicians can make sound management decisions.

Lucy Greig has been practising as a speech–language therapist in the
field of acquired swallowing and communication disorders for
over 15 years. She is currently the Clinical Director of the Rose

Rehabilitation Clinics at the University of Canterbury Rose Centre for Stroke Recovery and Research, providing diagnostic assessment and intensive rehabilitation to those with acquired dysphagia and language disorders.

Maggie-Lee Huckabee, PhD, worked clinically for 15 years before returning to university for a research degree. She is now a Professor in the Department of Communication Disorders, the University of Canterbury and Director of the Rose Centre for Stroke Recovery and Research at St Georges Medical Centre in Christchurch New Zealand. Her research interests focus on the complexities of behaviourally driven neural adaptation and biomechanical change leading to swallowing recovery.

Emilia Michou is currently an Assistant Professor of Speech & Language Therapy in Greece, and an honorary Research Fellow at the Centre for Gastrointestinal Sciences within the School of Medical Sciences, University of Manchester, UK. In recent years, she received independent research awards and funding from a number of sources including Parkinson's UK and the National Institute for Health Research (NIHR). In addition to research on neurorehabilitation of dysphagia, she teaches and supervises graduates and postgraduate students in the field of deglutition and its disorders, and continues to practise as a clinician. Dr Michou has recently been elected as a board member of International Association of Logopedics and Phoniatrics (IALP) and is a Vice-President of the European Society for Swallowing Disorders (ESSD).

Joseph Murray is Chief of the Audiology Speech Pathology Service for the VA Ann Arbor Healthcare System and an American Speech and Hearing Association Fellow. His research and publications are in the area of assessment, treatment and management of patients with dysphagia. He has focused his career on designing and delivering instruction materials in the area of dysphagia assessment.

Paige Nalipinski has worked in the Speech, Language and Swallowing Disorders Department at Massachusetts General Hospital for 25 years and is an Adjunct Instructor in Communication Sciences & Disorders at the MGH Institute of Health Professions in Boston. She is a senior clinician and specializes in neurogenic communication disorders, particularly dysarthria and primary progressive aphasia. She also works on the MGH Multidisciplinary ALS/ Neuromuscular Team.

Vicky Nanousi is a registered clinical neuropsychologist practising as a clinician in Greece, and teaching graduate and postgraduate students in the field of language and neuropsychological dysfunctions as a result of brain disorders. She completed her doctoral studies at the University of Essex, UK, following receipt of a PhD Scholarship from the Hellenic State Scholarship Foundation (IKY) Greece.

Julie Regan has 17 years' clinical experience in the assessment and management of adult dysphagia in an acute hospital setting. Her interests include, but are not limited to, instrumental evaluation, neurogenic dysphagia and oesophageal swallowing disorders. She completed her PhD in the School of Medicine in Trinity College Dublin in 2013. Her PhD thesis was entitled 'Adaption of functional lumen imaging probe to evaluate the upper oesophageal sphincter in oropharyngeal dysphagia'. She is currently an Assistant Professor in Trinity College Dublin where she is involved in the coordination of the taught MSc programme in Dysphagia.

Justin Roe is Joint Head of the Department of Speech and Language Therapy at the Royal Marsden NHS Foundation Trust where he has worked since 2007. In addition, he is the Clinical Service Lead for Speech and Language Therapy at the National Centre for Airway Reconstruction at Imperial College Healthcare NHS Trust. He also holds an honorary academic appointment in the Department of Surgery and Cancer at Imperial College London. He was awarded his PhD by the Institute of Cancer Research in 2013. As well as his clinical and leadership roles, Justin continues to be actively involved in research studies in the fields of dysphagia, head and neck oncology, lung cancer and laryngology.

Stacey Sullivan has been working as a medical speech–language pathologist for the past 15 years. She is a member of the adult swallowing disorders team at Massachusetts General Hospital in Boston, with the designation of clinical scholar. She has a specialization in neurogenic swallowing disorders and works as a member of the MGH Multidisciplinary ALS/Neuromuscular team, and at the MGH Center of Excellence for Huntington's disease. Stacey also participates in research studies that analyse aspects of speech and swallowing in the Center for Rare Neurological Diseases at MGH.

Paige Thomas graduated with a Master's in Speech and Language Pathology from the University of Canterbury in 2015. She is currently a PhD candidate at the University of Canterbury Rose Centre for Stroke Recovery and Research, mentored by Maggie-Lee Huckabee.

The combined research and clinical focus of the Rose Centre gives Paige the opportunity to be involved in a variety of complex cases. Her research interests include best practice for the assessment and treatment of dysphagia in neurodegenerative populations.

Margaret Walshe, PhD, is an Associate Professor and Head of Department of Clinical Speech and Language Studies at Trinity College Dublin. She has over 30 years' clinical experience in swallowing disorders and was instrumental in establishing the first postgraduate courses in dysphagia in the Republic of Ireland. She is a Vice-President of the European Society for Swallowing Disorders. Her research interests are acquired neurological dysphagia, implementation science and evidence-based practice.

Preface

Dysphagia is complex, with a presentation that often seems rather one-dimensional in medical research that leans to a focus on physiology and pathophysiology. This bias often fails to address the impact of dysphagia that is often most salient to the patient—it can rob people of the pleasures of eating and drinking that are often taken for granted. Events that act as a medium for developing communication in young children, establishing and maintaining friendships as we age, and providing solace and comfort typically involve food and drink. These social occasions may no longer be easy or possible for the person with dysphagia, with further repercussions for the lives of family and friends. None the less, each person will experience dysphagia differently, and will require various different assessment and intervention approaches that are influenced by aetiology and presentation. As such, there is much that we can learn from individual patient case reports.

Clinical Cases in Dysphagia provides a unique opportunity for clinicians and students new to the area of dysphagia to gain insight into the unique and varied presentation and management of dysphagia across a range of different conditions.

The terms 'case report' and 'case presentation' are used judiciously in the text and Chapter 1 expands on this, distinguishing it from single case study research design, which is the focus of Chapter 10. The intervening chapters present eight cases drawn from the clinical practice of a wide range of international clinical researchers. These diverse cases are used to deliver key messages on aspects of dysphagia management. Each case provides a different perspective and is accompanied by online resources to enhance case reports.

As clinicians who also work in academic settings, we recognize the usefulness of case reports in clinical education, because they provide valuable insight into clinical decision-making processes, and reinforces the message that 'one size does not fit all'.

Abbreviations

AAC	augmentative and alternative communication
ACBE	active cycle breathing exercises
AD	Alzheimer's dementia
ALS	amyotrophic lateral sclerosis
ALS-FRS	ALS functional rating scale
AMR	alternating motion rates
BiPAP	bilevel positive airway pressure
BiSSKiT	Biofeedback in Strength and Skill Training software
BMI	body mass index
BOT	base of tongue
CARE	CAse REport
CDR	Clinical Dementia Rating
CI	confidence interval
CN	cranial nerve
COPD	chronic obstructive pulmonary disease
CRT	cough reflex test/chemoradiotherapy
CSE	clinical swallowing evaluation
CT	computed tomography
CTAR	chin tuck against resistance
DOSS	Dysphagia Outcome Severity Scale
EAT-10	Eating Assessment Tool 10
EBSL	extended-spectrum beta-lactamases
EMG	electromyography
EMST	expiratory muscle strength training
FEES	fibreoptic endoscopic evaluation of swallowing
FEV_1	forced expiratory volume (during the first second)
fMRI	functional magnetic resonance imaging
FOIS	Functional Oral Intake Scale
FTD	frontotemporal dementia

FVC	forced vital capacity
GCS	Glasgow Coma Scale
GOLD	Global Initiative for Chronic Obstructive Lung Disease
HADS	Hospital Anxiety and Depression Scale
HNC	head and neck cancer
HRM	high-resolution manometry
ICC	intra-class correlation coefficient
ICP	Intracranial pressure
IDDSI	International Dysphagia Diet Standardisation Initiative
IOPI	Iowa Oral Pressure Instrument
LBD	Lewy body dementia
LMN	lower motor neuron
MBS	Modified Borg Scale
MDT	multidisciplinary team
MMSE	Mini-Mental Status Examination
MRI	magnetic resonance imaging
NBM	nil by mouth
NCS	nerve conduction study
NHS	National Health Service
NICE	National Institute for Health and Care Excellence (in the UK)
NIV	non-invasive ventilation
NMES	neuromuscular electrical stimulation
OAVS	oculo-auriculovertebral spectrum—Goldenhar's syndrome
OT	occupational therapy/therapist
PALS	person/people with amyotrophic lateral sclerosis
PBA	pseudobulbar affect
PCF	peak cough flow
PCP	primary care physician
PD	Parkinson's disease
PEG	percutaneous endoscopic gastrostomy
PEP	positive end-expiratory pressure
PPW	posterior pharyngeal wall
PT	physiotherapy/physiotherapist
PwPD	person with Parkinson's disease
QoL	quality of life
RAD	radiation-associated dysphagia
RCT	randomized controlled trial
RLAS	Ranchos Los Amigos Scale

RN	registered nurse
RoBiNT	Risk of Bias in *n*-of-1 Trials
RSB	rapid shallow breathing
RT	respiratory therapy/therapist
SCC	squamous cell carcinoma
SCED	single case experimental design
SDQ	Swallowing Disturbance Questionnaire
sEMG	surface electromyography
SLT	speech and language therapy/therapist
SLP	speech–language pathology/pathologist
SMR	sequential motion rates
SSRD	single-subject research design
SWAL-QOL	Swallowing–Quality-of-Life
TBI	traumatic brain injury
TIA	transient ischaemic attack
TOMASS	Test of Masticating and Swallowing Solids
TSAH	traumatic subarachnoid hemorrhage
UES	upper (o)esophageal sphincter
UMN	upper motor neuron
VaD	vascular dementia
VFSS	videofluoroscopic swallowing study

1 Case reports in dysphagia

An introduction

Margaret Walshe and Maggie-Lee Huckabee

Introduction

In the perfect world of clinical service delivery, all of our practices for diagnosis and rehabilitation would be fully supported by multiple, high-level, randomized controlled trials with consequent systematic reviews to provide assurance of efficacy. But our clinical practices are far from perfect and our evidence is far from comprehensive. Most descriptions of evidence-based practice thus allow the '[integration of] individual clinical expertise with the best available external clinical evidence from systematic research' (Sackett et al. 1996, p. 71). The valuing of clinical expertise is never intended to negate the power of empirical research, but does honour contribution of even a single clinical observation to spark the motivation for further investigation. Without the initial insights offered by a single patient, our well-supported practices would never have emerged. Therefore, although considered the lowest level of evidence, the humble case report in some respects is the origin of new thinking.

The aim of this chapter is to clarify use of the term 'case report', describe various types of case reports and emphasize the importance of using these to advance our clinical knowledge and practice in dysphagia. We provide a proposed template for writing case reports and some advice on publishing these for dissemination.

Terminology

'Case study', 'case report', 'grand round', 'case series', 'clinical case description' are all used interchangeably in the literature essentially to describe the same thing. In this text we distinguish between case studies and case reports. In case reports, changes in outcomes or responses to intervention cannot be explicitly attributed to an intervention and there are no attempts to control for extraneous factors. Unlike case studies and '*n* of 1' single study designs, case reports tend not to be planned or controlled but are rather a description of events as they occurred, in order to make a specific point (see Lillie et al. 2011). Case studies and *n* of 1 trials are discussed further in Chapter 10 by Murray in this text, and the term 'single case study' is reserved for research that is consistent with the experimental *n* of 1 design.

Importance of case reports

Case reports are important. Packer (2017, p. 4) suggests that 'case reports are all about novelty, serendipity, new ideas, fresh hypotheses and therapeutic surprises. Rather than provide confirmation, they provide inspiration'. Case reports can be considered naturalistic in that they involve the examination or exploration of cases in natural real-life contexts. Thus, they are excellent reflections of patient care, describing unusual presentations or exploring management approaches in real-life contexts while providing insight into facets of intervention frequently missed in larger research studies and clinical trials. They reflect the typical working environment rather than that of a research laboratory. They help generate an in-depth understanding of a specific topic to create knowledge and inform patient management. Case reports are considered important in recognizing and describing new or rare conditions, diseases or manifestation of disorders. There are peer-reviewed journals that are devoted entirely to case reports. Some of these, for example, *Respiratory Medicine Case Reports, Case Reports in Neurological Medicine, Case Reports in Otolaryngology*, may be of particular relevance to clinicians working in dysphagia.

Case reports serve a number of purposes. They can be used to convey a key message for other clinicians encountering similar individuals. This may be to draw attention to incidents where dysphagia is an initial sign or symptom of a serious underlying condition that is not immediately obvious. One example is a case report by Simmons and Bursaw (2015) describing the unusual presentation of a 61-year-old man with acute-onset dysphagia and progressive neuropathology that were ultimately associated with lymphoma and treated accordingly. Prompt diagnosis of the lymphoma was critical to the patient's medical outcome. Case reports are also used to describe the presentation and management of dysphagia in rare conditions. Lewis et al. (2015) describe the assessment and management of dysphagia in a person with Eagle's syndrome, a rare condition associated with abnormal length and positioning of the styloid process.

Case reports can further provide an in-depth exploration of the intricacy and individuality of a particular case in a real-life context from multiple perspectives, helping inform policy development and/or to direct and change professional practice. They may be used to help other clinicians learn from the errors of the authors (Sanei-Moghaddam et al. 2013) or challenge myths in clinical practice.

Case reports have helped us build and expand theoretical models to explain phenomena. One example of this is in the field of aphasia where cognitive neuropsychological models of language impairment were tested and developed based on phenomena exposed through single cases of individuals with impaired function (Ellis et al. 1983).

Finally, case reports assist in academic teaching by contributing to problem-based education for health- and social care professionals. Coyle et al. (2007), for example, use three case reports exemplifying both common and unusual clinical dilemmas in dysphagia to illustrate the process of evidence-based clinical problem-solving.

Types of case reports

There are many different types of case report and these may vary from short notes or a brief commentary to a more detailed patient description. Case reports can be categorized as follows:

Instrumental case: here the individual described is acting as in 'instrument' and used to illustrate a particular point, perhaps to a target audience or to provide a focal point for discussion on a specific management approach. One example is description by Joshi et al. (2008) of a 46-year-old woman with dermatomyositis and dysphagia. The clinical case report is used to discuss the association between dysphagia and dermatomyositis, and the potential treatment options available. A further example is a case report by Garcia-Carretero et al. (2016) describing a case where dysphagia was the only sign of a brainstem stroke.

Collective case: this involves studying more than one case simultaneously or sequentially in an attempt to provide increased support for a particular argument or theory. One example may be Thompson-Henry and Braddock's (1995) use of five case reports to highlight the failure of the modified Evans blue dye test to detect aspiration in patients with tracheostomy. A more recent example is a description of a series of patients presenting with a previously undescribed abnormal pharyngeal motility pattern by

Huckabee et al. (2014). This report highlights the importance of extending diagnostic modalities and provides speculative discussion of the aetiology of this type of dysphagic presentation.

Evaluative case: this is used to illustrate how well some specific approach is working. This could, for example, be a team approach to management or an intervention approach that has worked effectively. Perhaps this approach has involved a change to some facet of a more traditional management approach. Case reports are useful to demonstrate the result of this change, which may be positive, negative or neutral.

Explanatory cases: these aim to provide a depth of understanding on a particular issue providing potential explanations of perhaps some paradoxical finding. For example, a person with Parkinson's disease comes to the clinic with no report of difficulty swallowing but has aspirated on a routine barium swallow performed to investigate oesophageal dysmotility. This person has no respiratory signs of aspiration. She later aspirates on videofluoroscopy but is not symptomatic for aspiration. The ensuing case report might propose a theoretical framework to explain this absence of respiratory symptoms of aspiration in the patient. This explanatory case report may argue that the videofluoroscopy is not representative of her swallow function, that she is very physically active and walks for an hour each day with excellent baseline expiratory function. These explanatory case reports provide an excellent starting point for further well-designed prospective research studies.

Reporting clinical cases

The reader is directed here to a useful text by Packer et al. (2017) on writing case reports. It is recommended that authors consider first why they are writing the case report. Is this an exploration of some specific issue in dysphagia, an evaluation of a specific management approach or an attempt to explain some clinical phenomenon? Having identified a suitable journal or 'home' for this case report, the next task is to amalgamate the data and write the report. Many journals also require a patient consent form if the person in the case report is readily identifiable. This must be obtained in advance of submitting the report for publication.

Gagnier et al. (2013, p. 223) suggest that 'case reports written without guidance from reporting standards are insufficiently rigorous to guide clinical practice or inform clinical study design'. There are reporting standards for most types of studies. Templates for these are published on the Equator Network (see www.equator-network.org). Case reports are no different. Some journals, such as the *British Medical Journal*, have specific guidelines on writing case reports. These must obviously be followed when submitting manuscripts to these journals. Many journals also require a patient consent form but all attempts to protect the person's identity must be made with no identifying information in the case report.

Most journals adhere to the CAse REport (CARE) reporting guidelines. These were developed to improve the quality of case reports so that they can be of greater use to clinicians, patients and researchers (see Gagnier et al. 2013). An adapted version of the template is provided in Table 1.1.

Table 1.1 CARE guidelines (adapted checklist for case reports in dysphagia)

1. Title	**'Case report' should be included in the title.** This makes it easy to identify in electronic database searches and for systematic reviews
2. Keywords	**Keywords.** These are typically limited from two to five words and are the important words and concepts relevant to the case report
3. Abstract	This should involve three key components: a. *Introduction*: what does this case add to the literature on dysphagia? b. *Case presentation*: main symptoms of the patient, main clinical findings, main diagnoses and interventions, main outcomes c. *Conclusion*: What are the main 'take-away' lessons from this case? There may be an imposed word limit on this from the publisher
4. Background	Provide a brief background summary of this individual case referencing the relevant medical literature
5. Patient information	CARE recommend three main categories here: a. *Demographic information* (e.g. age, gender, ethnicity, occupation). Date of birth, medical record numbers; other specific identifying information should not be included b. *Main symptoms of the patient* (chief complaints) c. *Relevant medical, family, and psychosocial history* including information on relevant comorbidities including past interventions and their outcomes

(continued)

Table 1.1 (continued)

6. Clinical findings	Describe the relevant physical examination findings such as dysphagia screening and clinical examinations
7. Timeline	These are the important dates and times relevant to this case report. They can be depicted in a table or figure
8. Diagnostic assessment	This section includes information on the following four areas, as relevant: a. *Diagnostic methods* (e.g. instrumental assessment findings, videofluoroscopy, manometry etc., laboratory tests, imaging, patient questionnaires) b. *Diagnostic challenges* (e.g. ability to comply with procedures, financial, language/cultural) c. *Diagnostic reasoning* including other diagnoses considered d. *Prognostic characteristics* where applicable
9. Therapeutic intervention	This section should describe three areas relevant to intervention: a. *Types of intervention delivered* (e.g. exercise, pharmacological, surgical, preventive, self-care) b. *Administration of intervention* (e.g. the dosage, strength, duration and who delivered the intervention) c. *Changes in intervention* with rationale
10. Follow-up and outcomes	This section should summarize the clinical course of all follow-up visits. It should include the following four areas as relevant: a. *Clinician- and patient-assessed outcomes* b. *Important follow-up test results* (positive or negative) c. *Intervention adherence and tolerability* (including how this was assessed) d. *Adverse and unanticipated events*
11. Discussion	This section should include four main areas: a. *Strengths and limitations* of the management of this individual b. *Relevant medical literature* c. *Rationale for conclusions* (including assessments of cause and effect) d. *Main 'take-away' key lessons* of this case report
12. Patient perspective	It is recommended that the individual patient should share his or her perspective or experience whenever possible
13. Informed consent	Informed consent should be required for publication and provided if requested

Conclusion

Finally, it would be short-sighted not to recognize some limitations of case reports. Patients are typically studied in an uncontrolled environment and there are many confounding variables that can affect outcomes and case presentation. Authors should therefore not attempt to generalize findings to other similar populations but rather provide direction for further exploration if required.

In conclusion, case reports are important sources of information for clinical practice and future research. The case reports in this textbook are predominantly instrumental and evaluative case reports, supplemented with online resources to achieve a greater depth of insight into the management of the person with dysphagia. Each case report conveys a specific message to the reader and we encourage readers to use these as a means of reflection on current and future dysphagia practice.

References

Coyle JL, Easterling C, Lefton-Greif M & Mackay L 2007, 'Evidence-based to reality-based dysphagia practice: three case studies', *The ASHA Leader*, 12(14), 10–32.

Ellis AE, Miller D & Sin G 1983, 'Wernicke's aphasia and normal language processing: A case study in cognitive neuropsychology', *Cognition*, 15(1–3) 111–144.

Gagnier JJ, Kienle G, Altman DG, Moher D, Sox H, Riley D & the CARE Group 2013, 'The CARE Guidelines: Consensus-based Clinical Case Reporting Guideline Development', *Global Advances in Health and Medicine*, 2(5), 38–43.

Garcia-Carretero R, Bruguera M, Rebollo-Aparicio N & Rodeles-Melero J 2016, 'Dysphagia and aspiration as the only manifestations of a stroke', *BMJ Case Reports*, published online 11 February,.

Huckabee ML, Lamvik K & Jones R 2014, 'Pharyngeal mis-sequencing in dysphagia: characteristics, rehabilitative response, and etiological speculation,' *Journal of Neurological Science*, 15(343), 153–158.

Joshi D, Mahmood R, Williams P & Kitchen P 2008, 'Dysphagia secondary to dermatomyositis treated successfully with intravenous immunoglobulin: a case report'. *International Archives of Medicine*, 1, 12.

Lewis V, Hoffman Ruddy B, Lehman J, Silverman E & Spector B 2015, 'Management of dysphagia post operatively in a case of Eagle's syndrome', *Case Reports in Otolaryngology*, Article ID 305736.

Lillie EO, Patay B, Diamant J, Issell B, Topol EJ & Schork NJ 2011, 'The n-of-1 clinical trial: the ultimate strategy for individualizing medicine?', *Personalized Medicine*, 8(2), 161–173.

Packer CD 2017, 'Introduction,' in: CD Packer, GN Berger, J Mookherjee (eds), *Writing Case Reports: A practical guide from conception through to publication*, Switzerland: Springer, pp. 1–7.

Packer CD, Berger GN & Mookherjee, J (eds) 2017, *Writing Case Reports: A practical guide from conception through to publication*. Switzerland: Springer.

Sackett DL, Rosenberg WM, Gray JA, Haynes RB & Richardson WS 1996, 'Evidence based medicine: what it is and what it isn't.' *BMJ*, 312(7023), 71–72.

Sanei-Moghaddam A, Kumar S, Jani P & Brieley C 2013, 'Cricopharyngeal myotomy for cricopharyngeus stricture in an inclusion body myositis patient with hiatus hernia: A learning experience', *BMJ Case Reports*, published online 22 January.

Simmons DB & Bursaw AW 2015, 'Lymphoma presenting as acute onset dysphagia', *Case Reports in Neurological Medicine*, article ID: 345121.

Thompson-Henry S & Braddock B 1995, 'The modified Evan's blue dye procedure fails to detect aspiration in the tracheostomized patient: five case reports', *Dysphagia*, 10(3), 172–174.

2 Instrumental assessment and skill-based dysphagia rehabilitation following stroke

Lucy Greig, Kristin Gozdzikowska and Maggie-Lee Huckabee

Introduction

In clinical practice, limited improvement following rehabilitation is routinely attributed to a poor prognosis or lack of efficacy of rehabilitation approaches. Indeed, a recent Cochrane review (n = 6779), reported that 'there remains insufficient data on the effect of swallowing therapy, feeding and nutritional and fluid supplementation on functional outcome and death in dysphagic patients with acute or subacute stroke' (Geeganage et al. 2012, p. 2). However, a rarely discussed reality may be that the underlying pathophysiology was misdiagnosed, through either clinician error or ignorance. This may be understandable given our rudimentary classification system of pathology in dysphagia (e.g. weakness; Huckabee & Macrae 2014). If we lack the tools or the depth of knowledge to identify pathophysiology with specificity, how can we then plan rehabilitation approaches that are efficacious? Perhaps our patients do not fail treatment, but we fail our patients by designing rehabilitation approach that are not specific to their impairment.

Videofluoroscopic swallowing study (VFSS) is largely considered the gold standard in evaluation of deglutition because it can visualize all stages of swallowing as an integrated process (Rugiu 2007) and has been utilized in research and clinical practice for over 40 years (Logemann et al. 1977). This instrumentation provides two-dimensional, dynamic, radiographic images of swallowing, allowing frame-by-frame analysis of ingestive biomechanics (Feinberg 1993). VFSS evaluates temporal characteristics of swallowing, including duration and onset of swallowing phases (Fox et al. 2014; Leonard et al. 2000, 2011), kinematic events (Bardan et al. 2006; Humbert et al. 2013; Macrae et al. 2014; Sia et al. 2012), integrity of airway protection (Feinberg 1993; Hind et al. 2009; Kelly et al. 2007; Robbins et al. 1999) and the effects of compensation (Baylow et al. 2009; Bülow et al.

1999, 2001, 2002). Despite the undisputed utility of VFSS, there are limitations. Researchers have highlighted pronounced concerns with regard to reliability in interpretation of VFSS. Ekberg et al. (1988) investigated the reliability of radiologists scoring VFSS. Although the highest reliability was found for identification of aspiration ($k = 0.83$), the lowest concurrence was for critical swallowing parameters such as decreased or absent pharyngeal constriction and delayed opening of the upper oesophageal sphincter (UES) ($k < 0.40$; Ekberg et al. 1988). Even in implementation of standard protocols, reliability has been found to be similarly poor ($k = 0.01–0.56$; Stoeckli et al. 2003). This poor agreement has been replicated with speech–language pathologists in similar studies (Kuhlemeier et al. 1998; Scott et al. 1998). In a recent systematic review, Baijens et al. (2013) reported 45 measurements in VFSS varied considerably with an intra-class correlation coefficient (ICC) between 0.22 and 0.84, depending on the method of measurement, pre-experimental training and bolus consistency used. Increases in inter-rater reliability to greater than 80% have been achieved with standard protocols, but these programmes require criterion-referenced training (Baijens et al. 2013; Martin-Harris et al. 2008).

Although undoubtedly a valuable tool for visualising swallowing biomechanics, the widespread dependence on VFSS in isolation may contribute to misdiagnosis in the evaluation of dysphagia. For example, weakness as a primary characteristic of dysphagia is thought to be readily identified on VFSS because the muscles in question visually present with reduced movement and force (Stierwalt & Youmans 2007). Importantly, however, a hypertonic muscle would be characterized by rigidity or increased tone, causing an inhibition of movement, which may appear radiographically similar to the lack of movement seen in weak, hypotonic muscles. Recently reported patients with pharyngeal mis-sequencing (Huckabee et al. 2014) presented with diffuse pharyngeal residue when swallowing, which is routinely mis-interpreted as a symptom of weakness. However, further investigation with pharyngeal manometry identified mis-sequenced timing of pressure generation in the pharynx, despite relatively normal magnitude of pressure generation. This highlights the limitation of VFSS which only shows biomechanical movement, but fails to identify the underlying neurophysiological abnormalities that impact that movement. Thus, the observation of movement, whether clinical or instrumental, is prone to bias by preconceived ideas, such as inferences of strength from subjective interpretation of two-dimensional movement on VFSS. There is a need for more objective adjuncts to make the current gold standard diagnostic imaging technique increasingly robust.

Pharyngeal manometry is the only method of quantifying pressure in the pharynx during swallowing. It has been used for more than 20 years to objectively evaluate numerous parameters of swallowing physiology (Castell & Castell 1993; Dodds et al. 1987). Despite this, pharyngeal manometry has been slow to emerge into routine clinical practice (Ravich 1995). In a recent survey of 206 speech–language pathologists, Jones et al. (2014) documented that only 3.5% of respondents reported having access to manometry in their workplace. This is compounded by the finding that, of those who had access to manometry, only half reported they would pursue further manometric evaluation in a case study of a patient presenting with UES dysfunction (Jones et al. 2014). This highlights the need for continued education with regard to the availability and indications for use of the various diagnostic techniques in the dysphagia armamentarium. Although manometric assessment cannot differentially diagnose the presence or absence of weakness that underlies decreased pressure, it can provide valuable information about the characteristics of pharyngeal pressure and the contribution of UES opening to bolus flow. The following case report discusses the importance of objective instrumental evaluation of swallowing, and repeat assessment when limited improvement occurs. It highlights the importance of asking the questions: Did my patient fail treatment? Or have I failed in diagnosis?

Presenting concerns

JD was a 70-year-old retired man, who was married with two children and four grandchildren. He enjoyed playing golf and sewing horse saddles. JD used bilevel positive airway pressure (BiPAP) at night for sleep apnoea and had a past medical history of hypothyroidism and mild hearing loss.

On 17 September 2016, he had a right posterior cerebral artery stroke. Magnetic resonance imaging (MRI) confirmed an acute right occipital lobe infarct, right posterolateral medullary infarct and old left posterior inferior cerebellar infarct. Thrombolysis was unsuccessful and two days later he developed severe type 2 respiratory failure secondary to aspiration of emesis arising from a small gastrointestinal bleed post-thrombolysis. JD was admitted to the intensive care unit and a tracheostomy was inserted on 29 September 2016 after failed extubation. Feeding initially commenced via a nasogastric tube with subsequent percutaneous endoscopic gastrostomy (PEG) tube placement on 3 November 2016.

An initial VFSS was conducted two months post-stroke, following decannulation, and while still in the inpatient ward. JD presented profound dysphagia, including inconsistent elicitation of pharyngeal swallowing, nasal redirection, absent epiglottic deflection and no transfer of contrast through the UES. As well, he presented intra- and post-swallow aspiration with a cough response. Of particular note, he was able to expectorate some pharyngeal residual into the mouth. On the recommendation of his acute hospital clinicians, JD commenced inpatient swallowing-strengthening exercises, including effortful swallow, chin tuck against resistance (CTAR), head lift, and soft palate strengthening exercises.

One month after this initial VFSS, JD was referred for a fibreoptic endoscopic evaluation of swallowing (FEES). JD was diagnosed with right vocal fold palsy. No apparent gains were observed in his swallowing despite the completion of his inpatient strengthening regimen. Saliva pooled in the pyriform fossa, right greater than left, and free aspiration of secretions was observed.

Four months post-stroke, JD was discharged from hospital, nil by mouth (NBM) with all nutrition via a PEG; he managed his saliva by expectorating into a cup. He was then referred to a specialist dysphagia rehabilitation and research centre for intensive rehabilitation of swallowing. The overall timeline for medical history and interventions is provided in Table 2.1.

Clinical findings

At the time of his outpatient referral for intensive treatment, JD was ambulatory with mild persisting ataxia. He was living in his home and well supported by his wife who accompanied him to treatment.

A clinical swallowing examination was completed, which included cranial nerve examination, cough reflex testing, observation of swallowing with thin fluid and two quality-of-life questionnaires. More advanced, quantitative, clinical assessment (Timed Water Swallowing Test, Test of Masticating and Swallowing Solids), as well as further instrumental assessments, was deferred given the severity of presentation on prior examination and behavioural observation on this examination.

Cranial nerve (CN) examination revealed: reduced jaw strength (V—trigeminal motor); difficulty initiating consistent swallowing (IX—glossopharyngeal motor); asymmetrical palatal elevation with markedly reduced elevation on phonation—vagus and pharyngeal plexus); and reduced tongue strength on right side (XII—hypoglossal motor). The facial nerve (VII) was judged to be within normal limits. This presentation of CN findings is not inconsistent with the presumption of weakness based on his VFSS findings. On cough reflex testing, JD presented with

Table 2.1 Timeline of relevant medical history and inpatient interventions

Dates	Relevant medical history and inpatient interventions
Sept 2016	Diagnosis of a right posterior cerebral artery stroke affecting the occipital lobe infarct, right posterolateral medullary region and documented history of a prior left posterior inferior cerebellar infarct
Nov 2016	Initial VFSS revealed profound oral, pharyngeal and crico-oesophageal phase dysphagia. Strengthening rehabilitation exercises were commenced, including effortful swallow, chin tuck against resistance (CTAR), Shaker and soft palate exercises
Dec 2016	A fibreoptic endoscopic evaluation of swallowing. The patient was diagnosed with right vocal fold palsy. No significant gains were observed in his swallowing despite the completion of his inpatient swallowing strengthening regimen. He was discharged from the hospital nil by mouth with alternate nutrition (PEG tube)

Dates	Summaries from initial and follow-up visits	Diagnostic testing	Interventions
Jan 2016–Feb 2017 Phase I: development of a consistent swallowing response	Referred for specialist dysphagia rehabilitation. Patient was nil by mouth. He managed his saliva by expectorating into a cup	Clinical swallowing evaluation: • Cranial nerve examination • Oral trials • Quality-of-life questionnaire	GOAL: consistent elicitation of pharyngeal response and improved control of submental muscles APPROACH: skill-based training using the BiSSkiT protocol: twice a day, five days per week for two weeks
Reassessment		• Percentage of swallowing attempts producing a pharyngeal response • Percentage of pharyngeal swallows with adequate precision to hit therapeutic 'target'	GOAL: increased temporal precision in pharyngeal pressure generation with increased amplitude of pharyngeal pressure

(continued)

Table 2.1 (continued)

Dates	Relevant medical history and inpatient interventions	
	• Manofluoroscopy	APPROACH: trial skill-training with manometry—failed due to catheter placement issues resulting from UES non-compliance
Feb 2017–June 2017 Phase II: collaboration with colleagues	Referral to otolaryngology	Bilateral vocal fold bowing and lateralization and a hypertonic UES were diagnosed	GOAL: evaluate and treat vocal fold closure and UES non-compliance to allow catheter placement for therapy APPROACH: hyaluronic acid injection to the vocal folds. Balloon dilatation of the UES
July 2017–Sept 2017 Phase III: intensive, skill-based rehabilitation	Two weeks post-dilatation, a repeat HRM assessment was conducted	High-resolution manometry (HRM) • UES resting pressures before and after swallowing were significantly reduced compared with pre-dilatation measures • However, significant decrease in intra-swallow UES nadir pressure • Peak-to-peak latency between the proximal and distal pharynx of 26 ms	Daily skill-based therapy (45 min/day, four to five times a week) using biofeedback to improve sequencing of pharyngeal pressures
Sept 2017 Phase IV: final outcome	Significant improvement in patient's functional swallowing: • Consuming regular fluids and three soft-moist meals a day • Chest status clear • Ability to manage secretions improved	

a weak but intact cough response to 0.6 mol/L citric acid nebulized via a facemask on two of two trials using a suppressed cough method, indicating intact sensory branch of the vagus nerve (Miles et al. 2013).

On oral trials of two sips of thin water, JD struggled to initiate swallowing, expectorating the bolus and coughing violently. On the EAT-10, a 10-item symptom-specific outcome measurement tool for swallowing, JD scored 32/40, indicating high concern with swallowing function. A total score of ≥3 may be indicative of reduced swallowing efficiency or safety. JD also reported a decreased quality of life on all subscales of The Swallowing Quality of Life Survey (SWAL-QOL), with the exception of sleep. Although no guidelines exist for normative scores, it has been suggested that a subscale score of <90 indicates a decrease in quality of life (Pinchot et al. 2012). JD scored 0 on both burden and social subscales, and 18.5 and 25 on fear and mental health subscales, respectively, illustrating the significant impact his swallowing impairment was having on his quality of life.

Diagnostic focus and assessment

Phase 1: development of a consistent swallowing response

VFSS had been undertaken two months previously. This was not initially repeated because there had been limited symptomatic improvement and no reported clinical change in swallowing performance on FEES one month later, and swallowing elicitation frequency was low. Although his CN exam and behavioural assessment were not inconsistent with weakness as an underlying aetiology, strength-based rehabilitation had not been effective. In addition, a presentation of nasal redirection, paired with a site of lesion in the brainstem, raised concerns that the primary deficit may not be weakness, but rather a deficit of motor planning for swallowing. Importantly, adverse effects have been reported with strengthening exercises, such as effortful swallowing (Garcia et al. 2004) and current research is highlighting improvements based on skill, rather than strength, training (Athukorala et al. 2014; Humbert & German 2013). Thus, skill-based rehabilitation for oropharyngeal dysphagia was undertaken to improve volitional control of swallowing elicitation and improve precision in motor control of timing and relative strength of swallowing.

The initial focus of therapy utilized the skill-based rehabilitation protocol in the Biofeedback in Strength and Skill Training (BiSSkiT) software, with surface electromyography (sEMG) of the floor of mouth muscle represented by the software as a time by amplitude waveform.

JD participated in 20 hours (two one-hour sessions each day, five days a week, for two weeks) of swallowing skill training. Goals were to elicit a pharyngeal swallow every 30 seconds and to improve precision of voluntary submental muscle contraction during swallowing in both the temporal and the amplitude domains. Outcomes were measured by the percentage of swallowing attempts in which a pharyngeal response was produced and the precision with which JD could control muscle contraction during swallowing to successfully hit a 'target' on the screen with the sEMG waveform.

Reassessment

Success in eliciting a volitional swallow within a 30-second screen sweep improved from 33% of trials to 77% of trials over the two-week therapy block. The percentage of swallows with the peak of the waveform within the target box, a measure of precision in volitional swallowing movements, ranged from 58% of trials to 100% of trials.

At the completion of phase 1 therapy, JD reported that he was expectorating less saliva and mucus. Swallowing physiology was assessed using concurrent VFSS and high-resolution pharyngeal manometry (HRM) (Figure 2.1). Termed 'manofluoroscopy', this approach was used to assess the biomechanical and pressure aspects of JD's swallowing with

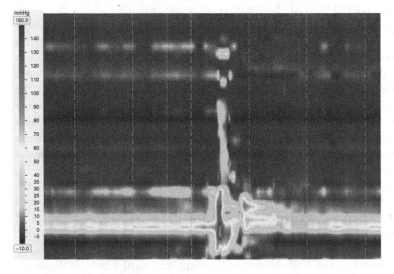

Figure 2.1 High-resolution manometry (HRM) spatiotemporal plot on admission

high temporal resolution, and objectively differentiate the aetiology of pharyngeal residue and restricted bolus flow through the UES. Specifically, the aim was to determine if the residual was due to diffuse impaired pharyngeal motility, pharyngeal dyscoordination or specific cricopharyngeal non-compliance.

At this reassessment, JD presented with mild oral phase dysphagia characterized by reduced lingual control, resulting in segmented anterior–posterior transfer of the puree bolus before swallow initiation and intermittent mild oral-transit phase dysphagia characterized by a mild delay (1–3 seconds) in initiation of swallowing after propulsion of the bolus from the oral cavity. As well, continued severe–profound pharyngeal phase dysphagia was evident with reduced velopharyngeal pressure (59.8 mmHg compared with a normative range of 154±42 mmHg—Mielens et al. 2011), minimal base of tongue-to-posterior pharyngeal wall approximation, with corresponding markedly reduced pharyngeal pressures (50 mmHg compared with a normative range of 307±172 mmHg—Mielens et al. 2011). In addition, there was minimal anterior hyoid movement with minimal/absent epiglottic deflection, diffuse pharyngeal residue, with 95–100% of the bolus subjectively judged to be remaining in the pharynx, and intra-swallow nasal redirection of the bolus (see Suppl 2.1—VFSS: mid-treatment). Of particular note, pressure within the pharynx was generated almost simultaneously in the proximal and distal pharynx latency within 15 ms, lacking the characteristic pressure sequence required for bolus propulsion. This is consistent with prior reports from a patient cohort with pharyngeal mis-sequencing, who had an average peak-to-peak latency between pressures at the upper to lower pharynx of 15 ms (95% confidence interval [CI] –2 to 33 ms—Huckabee et al. 2014). This is substantially outside on the 95% confidence interval from normative data (239 ms, 95% CI 215–263 ms; Lamvik et al. 2014). JD also presented with severe–profound crico-oesophageal abnormalities, characterized by limited UES opening, resulting in a post-swallow residue that filled the pyriform fossa. UES nadir pressure was 26.7 mmHg (normative range of –4±7 mmHg—Mielens et al. 2011).

There was frank post-swallow aspiration below the level of the vocal folds with thin fluids. JD had a strong cough response to the aspiration but this was ineffective in clearing the aspirated material. JD was sensate to pharyngeal residue; however, multiple dry swallows did not facilitate further transfer of the bolus into the oesophagus. Volitional pharyngeal expectoration was effective in moving some of the pharyngeal residue but was ineffective in moving the majority from the pyriform fossa.

Overall, JD's dysphagic presentation was multifactorial. He presented characteristics of weakness, consistent with CN findings, but these were compounded by generation of poorly sequenced pharyngeal pressure. This is consistent with a previously identified swallowing impairment termed 'pharyngeal mis-sequencing', characterized by dyscoordinated bolus transfer, intra-swallow nasal redirection and post-swallow residue (Huckabee et al. 2014). Finally, the influence of a non-compliant cricopharyngeus cannot be overlooked. This pathophysiological feature may also result in pharyngeal residual.

Phase 2: collaboration with colleagues

Based on this assessment, even though pharyngeal pressures were reduced, concerns about using strength-based treatment approaches were magnified, given the apparent absence of a temporally progressive pressure sequence and the presence of nasal redirection. Past reports of this presentation report that poor pharyngeal timing are exacerbated by effortful-type swallowing (Huckabee et al. 2014). To target greater specificity in rehabilitation, it was recommended that the focus of skill-based training shift away from the more general control of swallowing using submental sEMG. This would be replaced by a more specific control of increasing amplitude of pharyngeal pressure, while refining the temporal sequence of pressure generation, using manometry as a biofeedback device. Unfortunately, difficulty passing a manometry catheter through the UES made this approach challenging; therefore, after a brief and failed therapeutic trial, JD was referred to an otolaryngologist for evaluation and possible dilatation of the cricopharyngeus muscle. Bilateral vocal fold bowing and lateralization and a non-compliant UES were diagnosed. Medical intervention consequently included bilateral vocal fold injections with hyaluronic acid to increase the bulk and function of the vocal fold and balloon dilatation of the UES.

Therapeutic focus and assessment

Phase 3: intensive, skill-based rehabilitation

Two weeks post-dilatation, a repeat HRM assessment was conducted. The manometry catheter passed through the UES without difficulty. UES resting pressure was significantly reduced compared with pre-dilatation measures (23.9 mmHg and 46.6 mmHg, respectively), whereas intra-swallow nadir pressure remained within a similar range 25.8 mmHg (pre-dilatation UES nadir of 26.7 mmHg).

The dilatation therefore appeared to have improved JD's resting UES pressure but did not generalize to an improvement in intra-swallow UES nadir pressure. Pharyngeal manometry also continued to identify poorly sequenced timing of pressure generation in the pharynx, with a peak-to-peak latency between the proximal and distal pharynx of 26 ms, which could probably contribute to his intra-swallow UES dysfunction.

A daily skill-based therapy programme using HRM biofeedback was planned to improve sequencing of pharyngeal pressures while carefully increasing magnitude of pressure, and decreasing UES nadir pressure during swallowing. During treatment, JD was instructed to look at the visual biofeedback provided by the spatiotemporal HRM plot and swallow every 30–60 seconds (approximately one swallow per 30-second screen). During these swallowing attempts, he was instructed to inhibit simultaneous pressure generation in the pharynx, by changing the slope of the colour band associated with pharyngeal swallowing pressures. In other words, he was instructed to change the vertical line of pressure leading to the slightly lowered UES pressure (as seen in Figure 2.1) to represent a superior to inferior, left to right slope that terminates with the onset of UES pressure after relaxation in the UES (as seen in Figure 2.2). To prolong UES opening, he was instructed to increase duration of the low-pressure (blue) gap between the resting pressure (yellow–green) of the UES during swallowing. Finally, he was to attempt to increase the amplitude of pharyngeal pressure by adjusting the colour of the display *without* compromising temporal characteristics. Verbal and visual prompts and visual imagery were used continuously throughout the block of therapy. Baseline and post-treatment session measures of pressure amplitude and duration at the velopharynx, tongue base and UES on five saliva swallows without the use of biofeedback were recorded.

Follow-up and outcomes

Post-therapy assessment included HRM with impedance and VFSS (see Suppl 2.2—VFSS: post-treatment). As illustrated in Figure 2.2, JD could achieve sequential pharyngeal pressures when swallowing.

Pharyngeal pressures at the base of tongue increased significantly from 46.4 mmHg to 126.4 mmHg when swallowing a puree bolus, and from 53.8 mmHg to 92.0 mmHg when swallowing a 5-ml bolus of thin fluid. UES nadir pressure was within functional values when

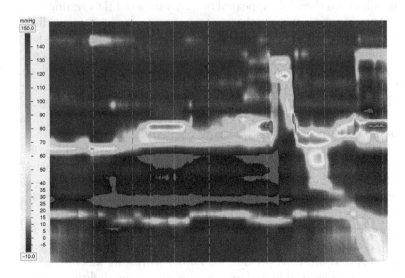

Figure 2.2 High-resolution manometry (HRM) spatiotemporal plot on
discharge

swallowing 5 ml of thin fluids and had improved for puree bolus (from
an initial UES nadir of 42.6 mmHg to 27.2 mmHg). With regard to the
timing of his pharyngeal pressure, his peak-to-peak latency improved
from 15 ms to 100 ms, consistent with similar post-rehabilitative outcomes reported in a cohort of patients with pharyngeal mis-sequencing
(Huckabee et al. 2014).

There was an associated and significant improvement in JD's functional swallowing and self-rated quality of life. Within 3 months of
initiating this treatment approach, JD is now having thin fluids and three
soft-moist meals a day. Nutrition through his PEG tube has reduced
to two supplemental Fortisips per day with a goal of discontinuing
tube feedings when fully transitioned to consistent and nutritionally
adequate oral intake. His ability to manage is own secretions has
also improved significantly. He only occasionally expectorates into a
cup when he is concentrating on a task and forgets to swallow. His
chest status has remained stable since the introduction of oral intake.
Importantly, JD's functional swallowing improvements correspond
with a significant improvement in both self-perceived dysphagia symptoms on the EAT-10 scale, with a decrease in total score from 32/40 to
11/40. JD reported increased confidence to try different textures/foods
and has been to a café for the first time since his stroke.

Discussion

Management of this patient highlights several issues that are of clinical significance. Based on CN presentation and VFSS findings, it was easy, and perhaps not inappropriate, to initially suspect weakness as an underlying aetiology of dysphagic presentation. Red flags of nasal redirection, brainstem site of lesion and difficulty initiating a pharyngeal response might have suggested other influences on biomechanics. Indeed, a muscle-strengthening approach did not result in functional improvement in swallowing. A consequent treatment trial using a general skill-training approach, which focused on volitional elicitation of a pharyngeal response, produced some positive effects; primarily he was able to produce more consistent swallowing on command. When further evaluation with manofluoroscopy identified UES non-compliance and a lack of sequential pressure generation, the treatment approach was adjusted to accommodate these more specific concerns. Medical management addressed the non-compliant UES. With greater UES compliance, the motor plan associated with sequencing of pharyngeal pressure generation become more obvious. The final treatment approach focused specifically on this abnormality using manometry as a biofeedback modality. It is clear from this case report, that repeated and/or varied instrumental assessment and biofeedback modalities were required to identify rehabilitation pathophysiology.

Use of biofeedback and intensity of treatment were key elements of this rehabilitation paradigm. It is well documented that biofeedback probably plays a critical role in the ability to maximize cortical capacity to modulate aspects of pharyngeal swallowing (Groher 2000; Humbert & Joel 2012; Lamvik et al. 2015). Further, intensive rehabilitation utilizes the principles of neural plasticity (Kleim & Jones 2008; Murray et al. 2003; Robbins et al. 2008). A systematic review revealed that intensive multidisciplinary rehabilitation was associated with reduced odds of mortality (odds ratio 0.66), institutionalization (odds ratio 0.70) and dependency (odds ratio 0.65) (Langhorne & Duncan 2001). Despite this evidence, McNaughton et al. (2014) revealed only 50% of rehabilitation units in New Zealand and 51% of rehabilitation units in Australia achieved 1 hour per weekday of direct therapist–patient contact time and state: 'few services in New Zealand provide community or outpatient rehabilitation more than 2 or 3 days per week' (McNaughton et al. 2014, p. 17). This is in stark contrast to evidence-based recommendations for rehabilitation to have a minimum intensity of 45 min/day, for each discipline. The present rehabilitation was conducted for 45 min/day, five days per week until optimal gains had been achieved. Therapy was conducted using saliva swallowing and swallowing ½ teaspoons of smooth puree bolus. Six weeks into phase 4 therapy, thin fluid was introduced.

In order to optimize best practice with regard to the evaluation and rehabilitation of dysphagia, a clear understanding of gaps in our knowledge and clinical methodology is needed. For example, broader understandings of unique patient presentations are difficult because many temporal parameters of pharyngeal swallowing are not easily observable on routinely used instrumental assessments due to inadequate temporal resolution. The onus is on the clinician to rethink and review rehabilitation options in the case of limited response to treatment, in order to avoid discharging patients on a modified diet or, even more significantly, NBM. Research indicates that patients who rely on alternative routes for nutrition and hydration at discharge from rehabilitation have increased risk of mortality at follow-up compared with those patients eating an oral diet or who had no signs of aspiration on VFSS (Ickenstein et al. 2005). Given these substantial consequences, when a patient fails treatment, the clinician should always first ask 'What have I missed?' before presuming that rehabilitation is not an option.

References

Athukorala RP, Jones RD, Sella O & Huckabee ML. 2014, 'Skill training for swallowing rehabilitation in patients with Parkinson's disease', *Archives of Physical Medicine and Rehabilitation*, 95(7), 1374–82.

Baijens L, Barikroo A & Pilz W. 2013, 'Intrarater and interrater reliability for measurements in videofluoroscopy of swallowing', *European Journal of Radiology*, 82(10), 1683–95.

Bardan E, Kern M, Arndorfer RC, Hofmann C & Shaker R. 2006, 'Effect of aging on bolus kinematics during the pharyngeal phase of swallowing', *American Journal of Physiology. Gastrointestinal and Liver Physiology*, 290(3), G458–65.

Baylow HE, Goldfarb R, Taveira CH & Steinberg RS. 2009, 'Accuracy of clinical judgment of the chin-down posture for dysphagia during the clinical/bedside assessment as corroborated by videofluoroscopy in adults with acute stroke', *Dysphagia*, 24(4), 423–33.

Bülow M, Olsson R, & Ekberg O. 1999, 'Videomanometric analysis of supraglottic swallow, effortful swallow, and chin tuck in healthy volunteers', *Dysphagia*, 14(2), 67–72.

Bülow M, Olsson R & Ekberg O. 2001, 'Videomanometric analysis of supraglottic swallow, effortful swallow, and chin tuck in patients with pharyngeal dysfunction', *Dysphagia*, 16(3), 190–5.

Bülow M, Olsson R & Ekberg O. 2002, 'Supraglottic swallow, effortful swallow, and chin tuck did not alter hypopharyngeal intrabolus pressure in patients with pharyngeal dysfunction', *Dysphagia*, 17(3), 197–201.

Castell JA & Castell DO. 1993, 'Modern solid state computerized manometry of the pharyngoesophageal segment', *Dysphagia*, 8, 270–5.

Dodds W, Kahrilas P, Dent J & Hogan W. 1987, 'Considerations about pharyngeal manometry', *Dysphagia*, 214, 209–14.

Ekberg O, Nylander G, Fork FT, Sjöberg S, Birch-Iensen M & Hillarp B. 1988, 'Interobserver variability in cineradiographic assessment of pharyngeal function during swallow', *Dysphagia*, 3(1), 46–8.

Feinberg M. 1993, 'Radiographic techniques and interpretation of abnormal swallowing in adult and elderly patients', *Dysphagia*, 358, 356–8.

Fox M, Pandolfino J, Sweis R et al. 2014, 'Inter-observer agreement for diagnostic classification of esophageal motility disorders defined in high-resolution manometry', *Diseases of the Esophagus*, 1–9.

Garcia J, Hakel M & Lazarus C. 2004, 'Unexpected consequence of effortful swallowing: case study report', *Journal of Medical Speech–Language Pathology*, 12(2), 59–66.

Geeganage C, Beavan J, Ellender S & Bath PMW. 2012, 'Interventions for dysphagia and nutritional support in acute and subacute stroke', *Cochrane Database of Systematic Reviews*, 10(10), CD000323.

Groher ME. 2000, Basic concepts of surface electromyographic biofeedback in the treatment of dysphagia: a tutorial, *American Journal of Speech Language Pathology*, 9, 116–25.

Hind JA, Gensler G, Brandt DK et al. 2009, 'Comparison of trained clinician ratings with expert ratings of aspiration on videofluoroscopic images from a randomized clinical trial', *Dysphagia*, 24(2), 211–17.

Huckabee ML & Macrae P. 2014, 'Rethinking rehab: skill-based training for swallowing impairment', *Perspectives on Swallowing and Swallowing Disorders (Dysphagia)*, 23(1), 46–53.

Huckabee ML, Lamvik K & Jones R. 2014, 'Pharyngeal mis-sequencing in dysphagia: Characteristics, rehabilitative response, and etiological speculation', *Journal of the Neurological Sciences*, 343(1–2), 153–8.

Humbert IA & German RZR. 2013, 'New directions for understanding neural control in swallowing: the potential and promise of motor learning', *Dysphagia*, 28(1), 1–10.

Humbert IA & Joel S. 2012, 'Tactile, gustatory, and visual biofeedback stimuli modulate neural substrates of deglutition', *NeuroImage*, 59(2), 1485–90.

Humbert IA, Christopherson H, Lokhande A et al. 2013, 'Human hyolaryngeal movements show adaptive motor learning during swallowing', *Dysphagia*, 28(2), 139–45.

Ickenstein GW, Stein J, Ambrosi D, Goldstein R, Horn M & Bogdahn U. 2005, 'Predictors of survival after severe dysphagic stroke', *Journal of Neurology*, 252(12), 1510–16.

Jones CA, Knigge MA & McCulloch TM. 2014, 'Speech pathologist practice patterns for evaluation and management of suspected cricopharyngeal dysfunction', *Dysphagia*, 29(3), 332–9.

Kelly AM, Drinnan MJ & Leslie P. 2007, 'Assessing penetration and aspiration: how do videofluoroscopy and fiberoptic endoscopic evaluation of swallowing compare?', *The Laryngoscope*, 117(10), 1723–7.

Kleim JA & Jones TA. 2008, 'Principles of experience-dependent neural plasticity: implications for rehabilitation after brain damage', *Journal of Speech, Language, and Hearing Research*, 51(1), S225–39.

Kuhlemeier KV, Yates P & Palmer JB. 1998, 'Intra- and interrater variation in the evaluation of videofluorographic swallowing studies', *Dysphagia*, 13(3), 142–7.

Lamvik K, Macrae P, Doeltgen S, Collings A & Huckabee ML. 2014, 'Normative data for pharyngeal pressure generation during saliva, bolus and effortful saliva swallowing across age and gender', *Speech, Language and Hearing*, 17(4), 210–15.

Lamvik K, Jones R, Sauer S, Erfmann K & Huckabee ML. 2015, 'The capacity for volitional control of pharyngeal swallowing in healthy adults', *Physiology & Behavior*, 152(Pt A), 257–63.

Langhorne P & Duncan P. 2001, 'Does the organization of postacute stroke care really matter?', *Stroke*, 32(1), 268–74.

Leonard R, Kendall KA, Mckenzie S, Ines Goncalves M & Walker A. 2000, 'Structural displacements in normal swallowing: a videofluoroscopic study', *Dysphagia*, 15(3), 146–52.

Leonard R, Rees CJ, Belafsky P & Allen J. 2011, 'Fluoroscopic surrogate for pharyngeal strength: the pharyngeal constriction ratio (PCR)', *Dysphagia*, 26(1), 13–17.

Logemann JA, Boshes B, Blonsky ER & Fisher HB. 1977, 'Speech and swallowing evaluation in the differential diagnosis of neurologic disease', *Neurologia*, 18(2–3 Suppl), 71–8.

Macrae P, Anderson C, Taylor-Kamara I & Humbert I. 2014, 'The effects of feedback on volitional manipulation of airway protection during swallowing', *Journal of Motor Behavior*, 46(2), 133–9.

McNaughton H, McRae A, Green G, Abernethy G & Gommans J. 2014, 'Stroke rehabilitation services in New Zealand: a survey of service configuration, capacity and guideline adherence', *New Zealand Medical Journal*, 127(1402), 10–19.

Martin-Harris B, Brodsky MB, Michel Y et al. 2008, 'MBS measurement tool for swallow impairment—MBSImp: establishing a standard', *Dysphagia*, 23(4), 392–405.

Mielens JD, Hoffman MR, Ciucci MR, Jiang JJ & McCulloch TM. 2011, 'Automated analysis of pharyngeal pressure data obtained with high-resolution manometry', *Dysphagia*, 26(1), 3–12.

Miles A, Zeng I, McLauchlan H & Huckabee ML. 2013, 'Cough reflex testing in dysphagia following stroke: a randomized controlled trial', *Journal of Clinical Medicine Research*, 5(3), 1–8.

Murray J, Ashworth R, Forster A & Young J. 2003, 'Developing a primary care-based stroke service: a review of the qualitative literature', *British Journal of General Practice*, 53(487), 137–42.

Pinchot SN, Youngwirth L, Rajamanickam V, Schaefer S, Sippel R & Chen H. 2012, 'Changes in swallowing-related quality of life after parathyroidectomy for hyperparathyroidism: a prospective cohort study', *The Oncologist*, 17(10), 1271–6.

Ravich W. 1995, 'The unrealized potential of pharyngeal manometry', *Dysphagia*, 43, 42–3.

Robbins J, Coyle J, Rosenbek J, Roecker E & Wood J. 1999, 'Differentiation of normal and abnormal airway protection during swallowing using the penetration-aspiration scale', *Dysphagia*, 14(4), 228–32.

Robbins J, Butler SG, Daniels SK et al. J 2008, 'Swallowing and dysphagia rehabilitation: translating principles of neural plasticity into clinically oriented evidence', *Journal of Speech, Language, and Hearing Research*, 51(1), S276–300

Rugiu MG. 2007, 'Role of videofluoroscopy in evaluation of neurologic dysphagia', *Acta Otorhinolaryngologica*, 27(6), 306–16.

Scott A, Perry A & Bench J. 1998, 'A study of interrater reliability when using videofluoroscopy as an assessment of swallowing', *Dysphagia*, 13(4), 223–7.

Sia I, Carvajal P, Carnaby-Mann GD & Crary M. 2012, 'Measurement of hyoid and laryngeal displacement in video fluoroscopic swallowing studies: variability, reliability, and measurement error', *Dysphagia*, 27(2), 192–7.

Stierwalt JAG & Youmans SR. 2007, 'Tongue measures in individuals with normal and impaired swallowing', *American Journal of Speech-Language Pathology*, 16(2), 148.

Stoeckli SJ, Huisman T, Seifert B & Martin-Harris BJW. 2003, 'Interrater reliability of videofluoroscopic swallow evaluation', *Dysphagia*, 18(1), 53–7.

3 Chronic dysphagia following traumatic brain injury

Julie Regan

Introduction

Definition of traumatic brain injury

Traumatic brain injury (TBI) is an acquired alteration in brain function caused by an external force (Maas et al. 2008). The European incidence of TBI is 235 per 100 000 (Tagliaferri et al. 2008). In the USA, the annual incidence of emergency room visits and hospital admissions for TBI are 403 and 85 per 100 000, respectively (Langlois et al. 2006). Common causes of TBI include falls, road traffic accidents, collisions, violent physical assaults, combat injuries and sporting accidents. Although the incidence of road traffic accident-related TBI is reducing with improved traffic safety laws, the ageing population is leading to increased fall-related TBIs. Better understanding of what happens to the brain after a TBI has improved its clinical management and hence mortality rates. Increased survival post-TBI poses significant costs internationally from medical, public health and societal perspectives.

TBI classifications (Figure 3.1)

The nature, intensity, duration and direction of the external force causing a TBI determine the nature and degree of brain damage. Primary damage includes diffuse axonal injury (multiple small lesions in white matter tracts), haematoma (solid swelling of clotted blood within the tissues) and contusion (bruising). Secondary damage can occur over hours and days and include inflammatory responses, ischaemia and raised intracranial pressure.

TBI has historically been classified as closed or penetrating, by clinical severity and by assessment of structural damage (i.e. neuroimaging) (Maas et al. 2008). TBI severity can be diagnosed using the Glasgow Coma Scale (GCS). This scale has three components (motor and verbal

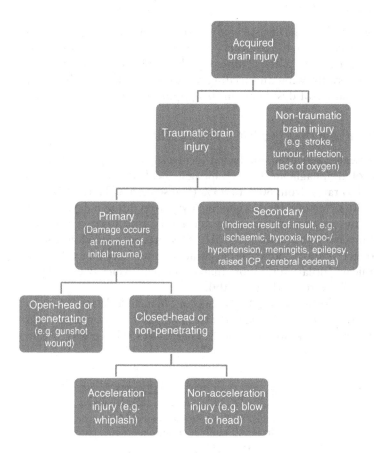

Figure 3.1 Traumatic brain injury classification

response, and eye opening), leading to a sum score of 15 (mild <13, moderate = 9–12, severe = 3–8). GCS scores can be influenced by sedation, ventilation, intoxication or paralysis. More emphasis has recently been placed on structural and functional neuroimaging, which are not affected by these factors. In the acute phase of a TBI, computed tomography (CT) examinations are carried out routinely in adults with a GCS of ≤14 or in those with a GCS of 15 who present with risk factors (e.g. vomiting, duration of amnesia, neurological deficit). The Marshall classification for TBI is a commonly used metric in acute care based on CT scan findings, which can predict outcome (Marshall et al. 1992). Magnetic resonance imaging (MRI) is more beneficial after the acute phase of recovery.

Signs and symptoms

TBI signs and symptoms vary considerably and can be categorized into physical, visual, auditory, neurobehavioral and cognitive–communication domains (Table 3.1). Each of these categories can impact on swallowing and feeding abilities, highlighting the multifactorial nature of dysphagia in this population.

Swallow dysfunction in adults following TBI

Little research has been conducted to investigate the prevalence and nature of dysphagia in TBI. Dysphagia incidence in TBI has been reported to range from 60% to 93% (Hansen 2008; Terre & Mearin 2009). Risk factors for developing dysphagia after a head injury include the severity of the injury on a CT scan, lower GCS score and Rancho Los Amigos Scale (RLAS) score on admission, abnormal tongue control, presence of a tracheostomy, feeding tubes and mechanical ventilation for more than two weeks (Mackay et al. 1999; Ward 2007; Terre & Mearin 2009).

Features of oropharyngeal dysphagia in TBI include delayed or absent swallow reflex, reduced tongue control, impaired hyolaryngeal excursion and silent aspiration (Lazarus & Logemann 1987; Terre & Mearin

Table 3.1 Traumatic brain injury (TBI) signs and symptoms

Physical	Changed level of consciousness, seizures, headaches, dizziness, nausea, vomiting; fatigue, paresis/paralysis, ataxia, apraxia
Visual	Changes in visual acuity, diplopia, problems with visual convergence and accommodation, photosensitivity, visual field deficits/visual neglect
Auditory	Outer ear, middle-ear and/or inner ear injuries; temporal lobe lesions; central auditory dysfunction; difficulty hearing speech in noise; hearing loss; hyperacusis; tinnitus; dizziness, vertigo, and/or imbalance
Neurobehavioural	Affective changes; agitation; anxiety, depression; impulsivity; irritability; emotional lability, mood changes; excessive drowsiness; increased state of sensory sensitivity, hypervigilance
Cognitive communication	Reduced alertness, inattention, agitation, impulsivity, memory deficits. Impaired verbal and non-verbal communication and language

2007, 2009). Other features of dysphagia, which differ from general neurogenic dysphagia groups, include abnormal reflexes (e.g. tongue thrusting, tonic bite reflex), altered muscle tone, sensory deficits, lip pursing or retraction, and swallow apraxia. Cognitive and behavioural features such as limited alertness, inattention, impulsivity, agitation and memory deficits often compound mealtime difficulties and can impact on candidacy for instrumental evaluation and rehabilitation.

Dysphagia treatment in TBI

Despite the prevalence of dysphagia and its significant contributory factor to mortality and morbidity in adults with TBI (Ward et al. 2007), research to determine the benefit of dysphagia intervention in TBI is sparse. Chin tuck prevented aspiration in 50% of 30 adults with TBI during a videofluoroscopic swallowing study (VFSS) (Terre & Mearin 2012). Neuromuscular electrical stimulation (NMES) has also been investigated in a small cohort of adults with severe TBI with promising results (Terre & Mearin 2015). However, cognitive and behavioural deficits often seen in severe TBI may be contraindicated for application of postural changes and NMES, and individuals must be able to elicit a swallow to be considered for these interventions.

In severe TBI, multisensory stimulation is a frequent starting point to rehabilitation to optimize alertness and attention (Padilla & Domina 2016). This is based on the theory that limited sensation causes poor motor response to the bolus. Sensory stimulation programmes provide frequent and repetitive controlled exposure to tactile, gustatory, olfactory or auditory stimuli. Research suggests that sensory stimulation can increase cortical activity (Lannin et al. 2013). Other techniques to assist with attention and orientation include involving individuals with feeding to promote appropriate oral responses to the bolus (e.g. hand over hand), changes in positioning, intensive tactile and verbal cueing, and environmental changes (e.g. quiet background, food presentation).

Functional MRI (fMRI) studies have revealed the multiple areas in the cortex responsible for swallowing (Malandraki et al. 2011). Given the neurological damage imposed by a TBI, the cortical areas controlling swallowing may be altered or damaged. Neuroplasticity is the ability of the brain to reorganize itself to compensate for injury or damage. It can be promoted through both endogenous (release of nerve growth factor) and exogenous factors (sensory stimulation) (Padilla & Domina 2016). Muscle plasticity is the ability of a muscle to alter its structural and functional properties in accordance with the environmental demands imposed on it. Neuroplasticity and muscle plasticity therefore serve as a good basis for rehabilitation, as clinicians strive to promote neuroplastic and muscular changes in order to improve impairments such as disordered swallowing. At the outset of rehabilitation, principles of neuroplasticity help to gauge candidacy and tailor treatment (Kleim & Jones 2008; Robbins et al. 2008). These principles suggest that factors such as age, time since injury, as well as intensity and saliency of treatment impact on recovery.

Presenting concerns

Eileen is a 70-year-old woman who was referred to a hospital dysphagia clinic by a medical team in a residential care setting. Eileen is married and has two children who live nearby. Her interests included baking, dancing, music and gardening.

Clinical findings

Seven years before the referral, Eileen (age 63 years) fell in her garden, which led to a traumatic subarachnoid haemorrhage (TSAH). Based on her GCS score (8/15), Eileen presented with a severe head injury which impacted considerably on her neurological and cognitive status. She remained in hospital for seven weeks. Once she regained consciousness, she reacted to external stimuli inconsistently with limited responses (Rancho Los Amigos Scale, level 2). Neurobehavioral problems included flat affect and excessive drowsiness. She was transferred to a neurorehabilitation setting for three months where she did not benefit significantly from physical rehabilitation. Six months after her accident, she was moved to a residential care setting where she remains today.

Eileen reportedly had numerous clinical swallowing evaluations (CSEs) and a VFSS during her acute inpatient hospital stay after her TBI. She was deemed to have a severe dysphagia, with a score of 1 based on the Dysphagia Outcome and Severity Scale [DOSS] (O'Neil et al. 1999), with an inconsistent swallow response and was placed nil by mouth (NBM). A PEG tube was inserted soon after her TBI to meet her nutrition and hydration requirements. Over the seven-year period, Eileen's weight has remained stable at 50 kg (BMI 19.5). She experienced occasional lower respiratory tract infections, which have been linked to vomiting events and her PEG feed. The rate of her feed was adjusted four months previously and she has had no chest infections since this change. From a medication viewpoint, she is on 20 mg omeprazole.

Eileen has remained wheelchair bound since her accident, with no functional use of her upper or lower limbs. She is unable to communicate verbally, although she can vocalize, and communicate discomfort and pain. She maintains good eye contact and her facial expressions are appropriate. She smiles to familiar music and to her husband's voice. Her alertness levels fluctuate throughout the day.

Eileen received no active dysphagia rehabilitation over the seven-year period. This was reportedly due to her fluctuating alertness and a tonic bite reflex, which meant that she did not accept a bolus orally during CBEs. In addition, given the shortage of specialist TBI rehabilitation services, the presence of a PEG tube meant that she was not in urgent need of dysphagia treatment. Despite this, seven years on, Eileen's family pursued dysphagia rehabilitation because they believed that some form of oral intake could improve her quality of life. They requested that her medical team refer her to an external outpatient dysphagia clinic to ascertain if she might be suitable for swallow rehabilitation.

Clinical hypothesis based on presentation and research literature

Eileen presents with chronic severe dysphagia caused by her TBI seven years previously. Issues to consider include the time since her TBI because her likelihood to recover from a neuroplastic viewpoint

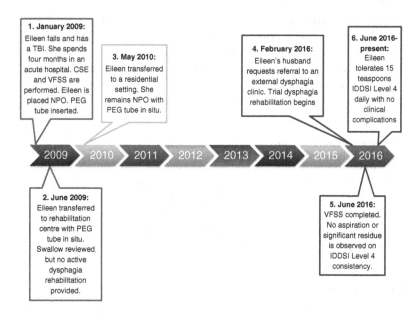

Figure 3.2 Timeline of clinical care

is uncertain. Also, the neuroplasticity principle of 'use it or lose it' suggests that her NPO status over this time period may have resulted in limited cortical reorganization for swallowing. In addition, as exercise-induced neuroplasticity occurs more readily in younger people, Eileen's age needs to be considered (Kleim & Jones 2008). Other issues are Eileen's fluctuating alertness both for rehabilitation and for mealtimes. Similarly, the presence of a tonic bite reflex may impact on her ability to accept a food bolus. Finally, Eileen's medical status, including her lack of mobility, her PEG feeding and her impaired cognition, makes her at high risk of an aspiration pneumonia. The introduction of any oral intake would need to be carefully considered by the multidisciplinary team.

Despite these potential barriers to recovery, Eileen and her family have not yet had the opportunity to avail themselves of a trial of intensive dysphagia rehabilitation over the seven-year time period. Eileen's husband reported that she really enjoyed food and baking before her accident. He suggested that the introduction of even small quantities of food would have a large impact on her quality of life, and it would give the family great pleasure in this chronic phase of her TBI to see her progress to a position where she could enjoy food.

Diagnostic focus and assessment

Eileen initially attended our clinic with her husband. She was wheelchair bound and had no functional upper or lower limb movement. Eileen had good eye contact and she exhibited appropriate facial expressions. She had no verbal communication. Occasional voicing was observed (e.g. when anxious). As Eileen was unable to complete motor responses to command, assessment findings were based mostly on observation.

Orofacial examination

She presented with right facial weakness and poor lip seal (cranial nerve [CN] VII motor). Some spontaneous saliva swallowing was observed. She was managing her saliva well, although a hyoscine patch was observed behind her left ear. From an airway protection perspective, she could produce strong vocalizations indicating that vocal folds were adducting to some degree.

Swallowing trial

Eileen could not self-feed but hand-over-hand assistance for feeding was feasible. She presented with a tonic bite reflex, defined as reflexive, sustained jaw closure, accompanied by increased abnormal tone in the jaw muscles, in response to stimulation. In Eileen's case, her bite reflex was in response to the sensation of an object on her lips. There was very limited mouth opening and teeth clenching in response to a spoon. Oral and pharyngeal phase of swallow could therefore not be evaluated. Some spontaneous saliva swallowing was observed and she did not present with sialorrhoea. Eileen therefore presented with severe dysphagia with a Functional Oral Intake Scale (FOIS) rating of 1 (Crary et al. 2005).

Instrumental examination

As Eileen was not accepting a bolus, a VFSS would not be of benefit. A fibreoptic endoscopic evaluation of swallowing (FEES) examination would have been beneficial to evaluate saliva management, pharyngeal structures and airway protection. However, based on a discussion with her husband, it was deemed unsuitable due to Eileen's cognition and anxiety.

Therapeutic focus and assessment

Based on this initial assessment, *exploratory dysphagia rehabilitation* was recommended. Treatment aims were to optimize alertness for feeding, minimize her tonic bite reflex, and provide sensory stimulation to improve the timing, safety and efficiency of her motor swallow response. Ultimately, the aim was to return Eileen to partial PO intake both (1) for quality of life and (2) to rehabilitate her swallow from a neuroplasticity viewpoint. In order to manage family members' expectations, it was stressed from the outset that a return to a full oral diet and/PEG removal was highly unlikely, given the extent and chronicity of Eileen's dysphagia, her fluctuating alertness levels and her risk factors for aspiration pneumonia. Her family understood this and were very agreeable to the proposed plan.

Eileen and her husband attended dysphagia rehabilitation sessions four times weekly (30-minute sessions) a three-month period. This intensity was required in order to induce any neuroplastic change. Sessions were scheduled for a time of day when Eileen was most alert. She was adequately alert for all but two sessions, when sessions were discontinued due to drowsiness. Rehabilitation is outlined in Table 3.2.

Follow-up and outcomes

After 12 weeks of dysphagia rehabilitation, Eileen attended a VFSS (see Suppl 3.1). She swallowed 18 teaspoons of sorbet, ice-cream and

Table 3.2 Dysphagia rehabilitation programme

	Rehabilitation	Aim	Outcome
Week 1	1. Multimodal sensory stimulation: Gustatory (sugar grains, salt, lemon, bitter administered by clinician to lips)	1. To increase alertness for feeding 2. To minimize tonic bite reflex	Increased alertness in response to music. Inconsistent and limited lip movement in response to taste stimuli
Week 2	Olfactory (containers of nutmeg, vanilla, herb mix positioned under nose by clinician)		Consistent lip smacking and inconsistent tongue movement. Tongue protrusion noted
Week 3	Auditory (familiar music such as Doris Day singing played in background during sessions, husband's verbal encouragement)		Client protruded tongue and introduced taste stimuli into oral cavity. She responded to taste stimuli appropriately (smiling in response to sugar and reacting strongly to salt and bitter). Swallow responses evident. Eileen's tonic bite reflex was markedly reduced and mouth opening was observed in response to stimulation
Week 4	1. Crushed ice introduced by clinician into client's oral cavity on a plastic spoon due to tonic bite reflex 2. Sensory stimulation (cold bolus, presence of spoon in oral cavity, auditory encouragement)	1. To induce neuroplastic and skeletal muscle recovery for swallowing 2. To improve quality of life	Client accepted the bolus into the oral cavity. Delayed oral onset noted before oral stage initiated. A prompt pharyngeal swallow noted subjectively. Anterior and superior hyolaryngeal excursion appeared evident subjectively Infrequent overt signs of aspiration (i.e. wet voice, reflexive cough, respiratory changes). Frequent liaison with Eileen's medical team ensured that her chest remained clear and she was not pyrexic

Week 6	Five plastic teaspoons of frozen (unmelted) vanilla ice-cream (International Dysphagia Diet Standardisation Initiative or IDDSI level 4). Eileen had previously enjoyed ice-cream and the temperature and taste was hypothesized to assist from a sensory stimulation perspective	She tolerated this small amount well at a slow rate and her enjoyment of this was very clearly evident (i.e. smiling facial expression. She opened her mouth in anticipation of the next bolus. No overt signs of aspiration were observed
Week 8	10 plastic teaspoons fruit sorbets (mango, raspberry, lemon sorbet) (IDDSI level 4)	Delayed oral onset. No overt signs of aspiration. This was considered an ideal bolus from a taste, temperature and consistency viewpoint. The rationale here was that swallowing small amounts orally will act as a rehabilitation to strengthen the client's swallow
Week 10-12	15–18 teaspoons sorbet (mango, raspberry, lemon sorbet flavours) (IDDSI level 4)	As above

food of puree consistency during the procedure. Findings included anterior spillage of material to the mid-chin during the oral phase of the swallow. There was a delay in the initiation of the oral stage of the swallow, which was aided by sensory stimulation (i.e. a cold bolus). The pharyngeal swallow was initiated at the level of the valleculae and efficient pharyngeal bolus clearance was observed. Hyolaryngeal excursion and upper oesophageal sphincter (UES) opening were adequate. Mild residue was noted post-swallow in the oral cavity and

Table 3.3 Outcome measurement

	Baseline	*Post-rehabilitation three months later*
Dysphagia severity (based on clinical swallow examination)	Functional Oral Intake Scale (FOIS) level 1	FOIS level 3
Oral intake	Nil by mouth	15 teaspoons International Dysphagia Diet Standardisation Initiative (IDDSI) level 4 daily
Instrumental examination	Unable to perform VFSS/FEES	DOSS level 2 based on VFSS
Chest status	Clear	Clear
Weight	50 kg	50 kg
SWAL–CARE (rated by husband)		
Goals of treatment for my swallowing problem	1	6
My treatment options	1	6
You had confidence in your swallowing clinicians	1	6
Your swallowing clinicians explained everything about your treatment to you	1	6
Your swallowing clinicians spent enough time with you	1	5

in the valleculae (Bolus Residue Scale = 2) (Rommel et al. 2015). She attempted to clear this without prompting. No aspiration was observed (Penetration–Aspiration Scale scores = 1) (Rosenbek et al. 1996). Eileen presented with a moderate-to-severe dysphagia (DOSS level 2; O'Neill et al. 1999) (Table 3.3).

The oral diet recommended for Eileen when she was medically well and sitting upright and alert were teaspoons of puree consistency (International Dysphagia Diet Standardization Initiative [IDDSI] level 4) food. Although the use of strong flavours and heightened temperatures was recommended, it was anticipated that other foods such as vegetables could be introduced with time. The limit of 15 teaspoons was to ensure Eileen did not become drowsy or fatigued during meals. Although, in the short term, it was recommended that Eileen was fed by a speech and language therapist (SLT) with her husband present for verbal cueing, her husband would be trained to assist with feeding in the longer term.

Update

Eighteen months later, Eileen continues to enjoy a limited oral diet on a daily basis. Her PEG feed remains in place. Her chest has remained clear. The introduction of oral intake has been a great source of enjoyment both for Eileen and for her family members. Her husband has received great pleasure in preparing food for his wife and in feeding her food she so clearly enjoys.

Discussion

Many individuals with chronic dysphagia are tube fed and deprived active dysphagia rehabilitation. This may be due to lack of evidence for dysphagia rehabilitation alongside the comorbid cognitive and behavioural issues that present in this population. In addition, lack of specialist rehabilitation services result in people with chronic dysphagia being nil by mouth unnecessarily. This case demonstrates that rehabilitation can benefit adults with chronic dysphagia post-TBI. The reintroduction of limited oral intake can have a significant impact on the quality of life of people with TBI and their families.

Patient perspective

Eileen's husband shared the views of her family throughout the seven years since her TBI:

It was very distressing for the family that Eileen was NIL by mouth for so many years. Her quality of life was shockingly diminished and being PEG-fed prevented access to neurorehabilitation therapies abroad. Without the expertise, dedication and friendly determination of the open-minded and progressive therapist, we would not have achieved the favourable outcome which helped develop and reactivate a swallow that had been inactive for several years. Eileen has enjoyed the swallowing exercises and the family has been overjoyed and inspired by this major advancement.

Bibliography

Crary MA, Carnaby-Mann GD, Groher ME. 2005, 'Initial psychometric assessment of a functional oral intake scale for dysphagia in stroke patients', *Archives of Physical Medicine & Rehabilitation*, 86, 1516–20.

Halper AS, Cherney LR, Cichowski MS & Zhang M. 1999, 'Dysphagia after head trauma: the effect of cognitive-communicative impairments on functional outcomes', *Journal of Head Trauma & Rehabilitation*, 14(5), 486–9.

Hansen TS, Engberg AW & Larsen K. 2008, 'Functional oral intake and time to reach unrestricted dieting for patients with traumatic brain injury', *Archives of Physical Medicine & Rehabilitation*, 89, 1556–62.

Kleim JA & Jones TA. 2008, 'Principles of experience dependent neural plasticity: implications for rehabilitation after brain damage', *Journal of Speech Language and Hearing Research*, 51, S225–39.

Langlois J, Rutland-Brown W & Wald M. 2006, 'The impact of TBI; a brief overview', *Journal of Head Trauma*, 21(5), 375–8.

Lannin NA, Cusick A, McLachlan R & Allaous J. 2013, 'Observed recovery sequence in neurobehavioral function after severe traumatic brain injury', *American Journal of Occupational Therapy*, 67, 543–9.

Lazarus C & Logemann JA. 1987, 'Swallowing disorders in closed head trauma patients', *Archives of Physical Medicine & Rehabilitation*, 68, 79–84.

Maas AI, Stocchetti N & Bullock R. 2008, 'Moderate and severe traumatic brain injury in adults', *Lancet Neurology*, 7, 728–41.

Mackay LE, Morgan AS & Bernstein BA. 1999, 'Swallowing disorders in severe brain injury: risk factors affecting return to oral intake', *Archives of Physical Medicine & Rehabilitation*, 80, 365–71.

McHorney CA, Robbins J, Lomax K et al. 2002, 'The SWAL-QOL and SWAL-CARE outcomes tool for oropharyngeal dysphagia in adults: III. Documentation of reliability and validity', *Dysphagia*, 17(2), 97–114.

Majdan M, Plancikova D, Brazinova A et al. 2016, 'Epidemiology of traumatic brain injuries in Europe: a cross-sectional analysis', *Lancet Public Health*, 1(2), e76–83.

Malandraki GA, Johnson S & Robbins J. 2011, 'Functional MRI of swallowing: from neurophysiology to neuroplasticity', *Head & Neck*, 33(S1), S14–20.

Mandaville A, Ray A, Robertson H, Foster C & Jesser C. 2014, 'A retrospective review of swallowing dysfunction in patients with severe traumatic brain injury', *Dysphagia*, 29(3), 310–18.

Marshall LF, Marshall SB, Klauber MR et al. 1992, 'The diagnosis of head injury requires a classification based on computed axial tomography', *Journal of Neurotrauma*, 9(suppl 1), S287–92.

O'Neil KH, Purdy M, Falk J & Gallo L. 1999, 'The dysphagia outcome and severity scale', *Dysphagia*, 14, 139–45.

Padilla R & Domina A. 2016, 'Effectiveness of sensory stimulation to improve arousal and alertness of people in a coma or persistent vegetative state after traumatic brain injury: a systematic review', *American Journal of Occupational Therapy*, 70(3), 7003180030p1–7003180030p8.

Robbins J, Butler SG, Daniels SK et al. 2008, 'Swallowing and dysphagia rehabilitation: translating principles of neural plasticity into clinically oriented evidence', *Journal of Speech Language and Hearing Research*, 51(1), S276–300.

Rommel N, Borgers C, Van Beckevoort D, Goeleven A, Dejaeger E & Omari TI. 2015, 'Bolus Residue Scale: An easy-to-use and reliable videofluoroscopic analysis tool to score bolus residue in patients with dysphagia', *International Journal of Otolaryngology*, Article ID 780197.

Rosenbek JC, Robbins JA, Roecker EB, Coyle JL & Wood JL. 1996, 'A penetration-aspiration scale', *Dysphagia*, 11, 93–8.

Taglaferri F, Compagnone C, Korsic M, Servadei F & Kraus J. 2006, 'A systematic review of brain injury epidemiology in Europe', *Acta Neurochirurgica (Wien)*, 148, 255–68.

Terre R & Mearin F. 2007, 'Prospective evaluation of oro-pharyngeal dysphagia after severe traumatic brain injury', *Brain Injury*, 21, 13–14.

Terre R & Mearin F. 2009, 'Evolution of tracheal aspiration in severe traumatic brain injury-related oropharyngeal dysphagia: 1-year longitudinal follow-up study', *Neurogastroenterology and Motility*, 21, 361–9.

Terre R & Mearin F. 2012, 'Effectiveness of chin-down posture to prevent tracheal aspiration in dysphagia secondary to acquired brain injury: a videofluoroscopy study', *Neurogastroenterology and Motility*, 24, 414–19.

Terré R & Mearin F. 2015, 'A randomized controlled study of neuromuscular electrical stimulation in oropharyngeal dysphagia secondary to acquired brain injury', *European Journal of Neurology*, 22, 687–e44.

Ward EC, Green K & Morton A-L. 2007, 'Patterns and predictors of swallowing resolution following adult traumatic brain injury', *Journal of Head Trauma and Rehabilitation*, 22(3), 184–91.

4 Management of a patient with amyotrophic lateral sclerosis

Focus on patient autonomy and quality of life

Paige Nalipinski and Stacey Sullivan

Introduction

Amyotrophic lateral sclerosis (ALS) is a motor neuron disease that is non-discriminatory in its reach. It prefers no singular ethnic, racial or socioeconomic group. When it strikes, life expectancy ranges from 2 years to 5 years from the time of diagnosis (Talbot, 2009). In that short period, all aspects of life are impacted. Initial symptoms can be quite different from patient to patient, with early symptoms, in retrospect, being subtle and gradual as muscles weaken progressively. There are two forms of ALS, sporadic and familial (genetic), the latter accounting for approximately 5–10% of cases in the USA (Valdmanis & Rouleau, 2008).

ALS involves degeneration of both upper motor neurons (UMNs) and lower motor neurons (LMNs). Patients who demonstrate UMN dysfunction may exhibit muscle stiffness or spasticity, slowness of movement, hypertonia, hyperreflexia, pseudobulbar signs and pathologic reflexes. Damage of the LMNs in the brainstem or spinal cord result in muscle atrophy, muscle weakness, hypotonia, fasciculations and diminished reflexes (Plowman, 2015). Patients may present with a combination of some, or all, symptoms.

In addition to motor symptoms, some individuals with ALS also develop cognitive changes. A large study conducted in 2002–2004 revealed that 50% of the patients with ALS present with cognitive changes and up to 15% of these patients met criteria for frontotemporal dementia (FTD), leading to behavioral and/or language impairment (Ringholz et al., 2005).

The speech–language pathologist (SLP) plays an integral role in the management of people with ALS (PALS) throughout the course of the disease. UMN and LMN damage can affect the bulbar region and impact both speech and swallowing function. Approximately 30% of ALS patients present with bulbar signs as the presenting issue

(Kiernan et al., 2011). It has been estimated that 95% of PALS will be unable to meet communication needs by using natural speech at some point during the disease progression (Beukelman et al., 2011), and 85% of PALS will experience dysphagia (Chen & Garrett, 2005).

Eating and speaking are our links to the world, and our connection to others. Shared mealtimes and conversations make us uniquely human. Loss of these abilities can be devastating, and threatening, to an individual's sense of self. The role of the SLP in working with PALS is to help them navigate the progressive loss of these functions in alignment with individual goals of care, with the aim of maintaining dignity and the ability to participate in relationships in a way that is meaningful for them.

In addition to dysphagia and dysarthria, patients with upper motor dysfunction may experience pseudobulbar affect (PBA), where they may laugh or cry suddenly and frequently, often out of proportion to the stimulus. Over 50% of patients with ALS experience PBA at some point. The prescription drug dextromethorphan has dramatically improved this symptom, and has had the benefit of improving speech and swallowing in many patients taking the drug. In a recent study by Smith et al. (2017, p. 770), it was found that dextromethorphan "enhanced speech and swallowing and improved the ability to handle oral secretions." The reason for this is not yet fully understood. Another option for pharmacological management of symptoms in ALS is riluzole (Rilutek), which is designed to slow the progression of ALS.

PALS are often seen in a multidisciplinary center where clinical experts help facilitate optimal care that addresses the complex needs associated with the disease. Research suggests that survival is improved when patients participate in this model of care (Traynor et al., 2003). During each visit, a patient will meet with a neurologist, registered nurse (RN), physiotherapist (PT), occupational therapist (OT), SLP and research coordinators, when appropriate. Also available to the patient may be a brace clinic, respiratory therapy (RT) and nutrition services, as needed (Paganoni et al., 2015).

The following case report describes the course of disease for patient WW (Table 4.1). WW has been living with ALS for over two years. He has generously offered to share his journey through his disease.

Presenting concerns

WW is a 64-year-old, right-handed man with a family history of ALS who presented in early 2016 with bilateral hand weakness, lower extremity cramps, and fasciculations, dysarthria and dysphonia.

I believe I first started experiencing symptoms in mid-2015 when I started experiencing severe cramping in my legs. I went to my PCP (primary care physician) in November 2015 for my general physical exam. I told him about the cramping but he brushed it off as age related. I asked him could it be ALS and he thought I was being alarmist because of my mother [who had ALS]. I knew I wasn't being an alarmist because the signs were there. The cramping in my legs was severe and my left hand was so much weaker than my right hand. Shortly after this I was noticing that my speech was slowing down somewhat, and asked to see him again. He looked at my hands and told me I should see a neurologist for an EMG (electromyography) exam. I had the EMG in February 2016. When they did my left arm and saw the results, they decided to do my whole body. The results were all abnormal and they said to me, "while I can't definitely say you have ALS, I'm pretty sure you have it." So, I came home and called the ALS clinic for an appointment.

Clinical findings

Past medical and surgical history

Lumbar spinal stenosis and degenerative spondylolisthesis, hyperlipidemia, hypertension and transient ischemic attack (TIA) with transient

Table 4.1 Timeline of relevant medical history and interventions

Date	Summary from initial evaluation	Diagnostic testing	Interventions
1/15	Night-time cramping in calves		
1/16	Decreased strength in left hand		
2/16	Hoarseness and slurring	EMG confirms denervation	
3/16	Decreased strength in right hand	Gene testing positive for C9orf72 gene	Start riluzole
4/16	Noted dysphagia	VFSS	Change diet consistencies
6/17	Worsening dysphagia	VFSS	
7/17	Pseudobulbar affect noted		Start dextromethorphan
7/17	Continued weight loss and worsening dysphagia		Gastrostomy tube placed

right hemiparesis (2006); medial right thigh glomus tumor resection (2010); L4–5 laminectomy/fusion with instrumentation (2013); lipoma removals from bilateral arms and chest (2016).

Family history

Mother diagnosed with ALS at age 61. His maternal first cousin diagnosed with ALS in her 50s.

Social history

WW lives with his wife in Massachusetts. They have two adult children. WW works as a social worker.

Neurological examination

Results of the initial neurological examination revealed mild weakness of the left arm/hand, diffuse fasciculations throughout the body and mild fasciculations of the tongue with trace impracision of his speech. There was brisk jaw jerk and frontal release signs. EMG and nerve conduction study (NCS) interpretation suggested motor neuron disease versus diffuse cervical polyradiculopathy.

Physical and occupation therapy examination

Results of initial physical and occupational therapy evaluations revealed little observable weakness in the lower extremities. The therapists provided education regarding management of stairs, modifications to the home for the future, and recommendations for moderate level exercises prescribed with fall prevention in mind. WW was encouraged to exercise strong muscles only, and not try to strengthen weak muscles, an approach that has been the focus of much research in the past decade (Lunetta et al., 2016). It was recommended that WW continue to work with an OT to address hand weakness causing difficulty with functional tasks (taking off socks, buttons, zippers, turning keys and lifting items overhead).

Scales and questionnaires [ALS functional rating scale or ALS-FRS (Brooks et al., 1996) and the ALS Severity Scale (Yorkston et al., 1993)], which are useful tools to measure change over time and to integrate patient perception into assessment findings and recommendations, were used during WW's visits.

Once I was diagnosed it was depressing, but I was introduced to several members of the team, and thought I had come to the right place. It appeared to me that all my needs, from OT to PT to speech therapy would all be addressed by the team and that gave me a feeling of comfort. I felt in good hands in the ALS clinic at the hospital and everyone was so caring and supportive.

Diagnostic focus and assessment

WW had a full neurological work-up largely to rule out other diagnoses, especially something treatable. According to the El Escorial Federation of Neurology (Ludolph et al., 2015), the diagnosis of ALS requires the presence of: signs of LMN degeneration by clinical, electrophysiological or neuropathological examination, signs of UMN degeneration by clinical examination, and progressive spread of signs within a region or to other regions, together with the absence of electrophysiological evidence of other disease processes that might explain the signs of LMN and/or UMN degenerations, and neuroimaging evidence of other disease processes that might explain the observed clinical and electrophysiological signs. WW's EMG in February 2016 confirmed denervation. At this time, he was prescribed riluzole in attempt to slow the progression of his disease.

Genetic testing in March 2016 via blood draw, found he was positive for *C9orf72*, one of two genes (the other being *SOD1*) associated with the familial component to the disease presentation. *C9orf72* mutation has also been linked to development of frontotemporal dementia (FTD).

Vital capacity testing was routinely conducted to measure ventilatory function. During the initial diagnostic visit his forced vital capacity (FVC) was 78% and in April 2017 was down to 72%, not a dramatic drop for a patient with ALS, although a marker of progression. This testing determines if interventions such as pressure support are needed for a patient. Some patients will require non-invasive ventilation (NIV), whereas others may require tracheotomy and ventilator support. In November 2016, WW reported orthopnea, dyspnea on exertion and with speech, and daytime fatigue, and NIV was initiated, though primarily just used overnight.

PT, OT, RT and SLP conducted assessments every 2–3 months to measure change and provide relevant recommendations for WW as his ALS progressed. Often, PALS are referred for short courses of therapy to maximize function dependent on the changes/decline identified during each assessment. This has been helpful for WW throughout the progression of his disease thus far.

An initial SLP assessment was completed in March 2016. WW was found to have intact tongue bulk, with no fasciculation or atrophy with tongue strength adequate for both lateral and anterior resistance. His buccal strength was within normal limits and he could maintain adequate lip seal during pressure to puffed cheeks. Palatal elevation was full and symmetric on phonation. His cough and throat clear were mildly weak without the power expected for his age and gender.

With regard to speech, WW's alternating motion rates (AMRs) (rapid production of reciprocal movements as in /papapa/) and sequential motion rates (SMRs) (moving rapidly from one articulatory position to another as in /pataka/) were both rapid and regular. His vocal quality was slightly strained and strangled, as well as hypophonic, and he was able to sustain phonation for 14 seconds, slightly below average of 15 seconds (Maslan et al., 2011).

In the office his swallow was assessed with water and cookies. He ingested water from an open cup. Following large consecutive cup sips of water, he had a dry cough for the remainder of the session. Oral preparation and transit of cookie bolus was prompt and complete, without oral residue. Throughout the session he was noted to breathe comfortably on room air. He did not appear to have any issues with secretion management, as there was no drooling or secretion pooling.

Overall, his initial SLP assessment revealed mild spastic dysarthria and symptoms suggestive of dysphagia. WW was referred for a videofluoroscopic swallowing study (VFSS) to objectively evaluate swallowing physiology and further guide diet recommendations and indications for postural maneuver/compensatory strategy use. A VFSS was completed a few days after the initial clinic visit, and revealed oral and base-of-tongue weakness that resulted in small amounts of residue in the vallecular space on completion of the initial swallow response. This residue was present for both liquid and solid bolus trials. There was penetration of thin liquid taken in consecutive cup sips and with a liquid wash to clear vallecular residue. WW was unable to maintain adequate glottic and supraglottic closure for rapid, repetitive bolus presentations. WW demonstrated improved bolus control with nectar liquid trials, because the pharyngeal swallowing response was more timely and the presence of penetration extinguished (when compared with thin liquids).

WW had repeated, abbreviated assessments from SLP in the clinic setting which included: oral motor and sensory examination, motor speech and voice assessment, swallowing and cognitive–linguistic screening. Based on the results of the clinic assessment, patients with ALS may be referred for formal cognitive and/or language evaluation, VFSS (to obtain objective information regarding swallowing physiology and aspiration risks), augmentative and alternative communication (AAC) assessment, and speech and/or swallow intervention.

By the end of April 2017, in the context of progressive weight loss and increased difficulty swallowing an oral diet, it was recommended that WW return for repeat VFSS to determine his ability to safely continue with oral nutrition/hydration and to help guide his decision regarding consideration of feeding tube placement. This swallowing study found a significant progression in his dysphagia, characterized by oral tongue, base of tongue and pharyngeal weakness, as well as delayed and incomplete laryngeal closure. WW demonstrated silent aspiration with thin and thickened liquid consistency during the swallow. Although not directly observed during this examination, WW was felt to be at significant risk for aspiration of post-swallow residue on completion of the swallow response. His diminished cough response was minimally effective to clear aspirated material. A chin-tuck strategy was found to be somewhat effective to improve airway protection and reduce post-swallow residue in the pharyngeal recesses. It was recommended that a gastrostomy tube be considered.

Although WW had features of spasticity in his presentation, he did not describe laryngospasm, an involuntary closure of the vocal folds that can be triggered by any stimulation to the larynx (penetration/aspiration of secretions, liquids, food particles, dust or even strong odors such as bleach). Typically, ALS patients with laryngopspasm experience a tight gasping rather than a cough, with the introduction of any trigger stimulant such as vinegar, red wine, etc. (Fourcade et al., 2010; Jackson et al., 2015). Providing PALS with education to help them understand the event and how to facilitate its passage (relaxation/breathing techniques) is an invaluable role of the SLT.

Therapeutic focus and assessment

In addition to specific diet modifications and postural maneuvers identified during the VFSS, WW was given recommendations regarding high-calorie, easy-to-swallow recipes for efficient calorie intake (ideally provided in concert with a clinical nutritionist), and energy conservation strategies that pertained to both swallowing and speech. He was also educated about simple speech devices he could use immediately such as a voice amplifier and text-to-speech applications for tablets and smart phones.

> As soon as it was recommended to thicken my drinks I started to do this. I had been having trouble with thin liquids, such as water and soda, causing me to cough and have trouble swallowing cleanly. This was around September 2016, four months post diagnosis. As my swallowing deteriorated, I had to modify my diet to eat foods that were processed through a food processor to make them easier to eat. My chewing was also deteriorating so

having my food pulverized and mixed in with gravy and sautéed vegetables that were processed became a necessity. It was easiest to swallow with my food pureed and allowed me to keep eating for several months and still enjoy food.

WW was familiar with ALS and its ravages, having watched his mother suffer with the disease. He was ready to hear and act on any suggestions provided during his visits. However, at the time of diagnosis, and during initial clinic visits, not all PALS are ready to consider the possibility that they may/will lose their voice and/or swallowing capacity. Based on previous exposure to disease and where they are in their grieving/acceptance process, patients process information very differently. It is important to give information early; however, it is imperative that the patient and family are ready to hear the information and are clear about their diagnosis and prognosis before a clinician attempt such education. Information delivery needs to be considered on a patient-by-patient basis; there is no one-size-fits-all guide to patient/family education and counseling. Social workers can provide invaluable support to patients and families throughout the course of the disease.

For WW, like many PALS, decision-making was at the center of his life and he was constantly negotiating with family and care providers at a pace that allowed him to "maintain a sense of self and wellbeing in the face of change" (King et al., 2009, p. 753).

I first remember talking with my mother in late 1978 when she told me she was having difficulty holding onto things and she actually dropped a plate in the kitchen. Later when she came to my social work graduation I have a picture of her with her hands curled in the fashion that I now know. Shortly after this in 1980, she was formally diagnosed with ALS. She began to lose her speech and she received an alphabet board, which she used to communicate. It was tedious spelling out whole words. Her progression with the illness was fairly quick.

WW and his wife were very proactive in their approach to disease management. Although motor speech and voice were quite functional at the time of initial SLP evaluation, they wanted exposure to all tools available that would help with communication in the future. WW was quite interested in message banking and AAC, so was referred for a full assessment at the time of his first visit. WW was interested in doing whatever it took to stay involved with his students and he knew that that meant embracing AAC early on (Costello, 2016).

Overall, my experience with the AAC program has been a good one. Initially when I first met the speech therapist and in the first session she showed me low-tech ways of helping me communicate with an alphabet board, I freaked. It was a bad memory of my mother brought right into the room.

Overall, I would say that I feel empowered by the alternative communication devices, and I am currently using one. They even encouraged me to "bank my voice" which I am using now. It is kind of weird to hear my voice from several months ago when I could still talk clearly and forcefully. The speech therapist has also shown me eye gaze software, which I will use when my hands no longer work. Even when I was still working at the school I began to use the Talk For Me software and I think the kids I work with all thought it was cool and it was a good life lesson in overcoming adversity. (Always the social worker.) I am grateful this type of technology exists now when it didn't for my mother. My wife and I can still communicate and speak to each other, and that is a win–win for me.

Follow-up and outcomes

Over the next 15 months, WW's dysphagia and dysarthria progressed. His mild spastic dysarthria had evolved with flaccid features, and he was no longer intelligible to unfamiliar listeners beyond short phrases. WW became increasingly dependent on AAC to interact with others.

As swallowing safety and efficiency continued to decline, WW was unable to maintain his weight and lost more than 20 pounds. Secretion management became a problem as well. A recommendation was made for use of an in–exsufflator (cough assist) and oral suction to assist with airway clearance. Medications were also often used to assist with secretion management (Jackson et al., 2015).

I began using the cough assist on a more regular basis and now use it every night in conjunction with the suction machine before bed. It works well to clean out my throat and allow me to breath cleaner and easier. I was also ordered glycopyrrolate for the control of secretions in my mouth. I now take this pill three times a day, and I feel it is quite helpful.

WW is seen in a multidisciplinary clinic every three months. During each visit, each member of the multidisciplinary team, including the

SLP, performs a reassessment of function, and provides supportive education and compensatory care. The entire team continues to provide education regarding the status of his progression, as well as address his wishes with regard to quality of life.

> Before the g-tube the doctors told my mother that she would die of malnutrition if she didn't do something. The decision to have a g-tube placed was compounded by my sister being pregnant and my mother wanting to see the baby born. My mother and I talked quite a bit about the g-tube and I actually advised against it. By this time, she was completely immobile and could no longer talk. Several times in spelling out words she asked me to help her die. I thought about it but decided I couldn't do that to my father who was devoted to her. She received little to no care from any hospital or doctors during this stage of the illness. She had to be suctioned out every day and the machines were archaic. She eventually lost the ability to blink her eyes and so couldn't communicate anymore. CW and I had met by this point. We planned our wedding in New York so my mother could attend but she died in March 1984 and we were married in May 1984. It was a relief that she died, peacefully on the couch. All told I think the g-tube stabilized her decline and afforded her 2 more years of a very horrible life.
>
> I was very mixed about the g-tube from the outset mainly because of my mother's experience with it. It was about 35 years ago that she had it placed and I have very bad memories about it. So all along this journey I thought I would never do the g-tube. I didn't want any advanced measures to keep me alive. But lately my swallowing has deteriorated so much that I can't survive without nutrition. I know my coughing and choking on food is very disturbing to my wife, so partly the g-tube is a way to reduce the hassle for us both.
>
> I have my family to think about. A new granddaughter, and my own children and wife who I am not yet ready to say goodbye to. I am accepting this g-tube now but I made CW promise when I say I am done she can't continue to feed me through it. I believe she will accept my wishes and do what I ask.
>
> With my legs still strong and working I've decided that the g-tube is preferential because I can't swallow and I'm not yet ready to give up and die. As far as a trach or vent, I will not go that route. When I can't breathe on my own, that's the end for me.

For PALS, placement of a tracheostomy with mechanical ventilation is a palliative option, with high quality of life expressed by patients, but with very high burden of care on care providers (Kaub-Wittemer et al., 2003). Life is prolonged, but patients require 24-hour care and the overall costs are exorbitant, approximately $199,500 per year (Obermann & Lyon, 2015). WW has made it clear that this is not the path he wished to take.

Closing statement from WW

> Life is never easy, even in the best of moments. It's in these moments of crisis that you find your inner reserves, the strength to go on even when to do so seems impossible. That is my task now. To not lose faith, to find wonderment in the smallest things, and to find love in my relationships with family and friends. This is my life now. I was busy making other plans, but now my vision is to surround myself with the people who love me the most.

Discussion

Bulbar signs impacting speech and swallowing can vary greatly among patients and may include articulatory imprecision and/or difficulty with oral manipulation of foods/liquids (tongue weakness or spasticity), hypernasality and/or nasal regurgitation (weakened soft palate), difficulty with bilabials and/or retention of food in the oral cavity lip weakness), slowed rate (spasticity in the whole bulbar system), changes in vocal quality (vocal fold weakness or spasticity) (Darley et al., 1969; Duffy, 2005; Kuhnlein et al., 2008; Tomik & Guiloff, 2010). Patients may have a weak, non-productive cough (weak respiratory system). The SLP plays a crucial role in helping patients live with these symptoms/deficits.

Patients with ALS face rapid and devastating declines in all aspects of their lives. Meaningful intervention by experienced professionals can help them manage symptoms, procure appropriate equipment in a timely manner and work with them to be sure that their goals of care are met. Medical treatments are minimal, but quality of life can be profoundly impacted if the patient faces the disease with a compassionate and knowledgeable team at his side.

References

Beukelman DR, Fagar S & Nordness A. 2011, 'Communication support for people with ALS,' *Neurology Research International*, article ID 714693.

Brooks B, Sanjak M et al. 1996, 'The amyotrophic lateral sclerosis functional rating scale—Assessment of activities of daily living in patients with amyotrophic lateral sclerosis', *Archives of Neurology*, 53(2), 141–7.

Chen A & Garrett CG 2005, 'Otolaryngologic presentations of amyotrophic lateral sclerosis', *Otolaryngology—Head and Neck Surgery*, 132(3), 500–4.

Costello J. 2016, 'Message banking vs. voice banking: a very successful proactive model for people with ALS/MND', paper presented at 14th Annual Allied Professionals Forum, International Alliance of ALS/MND Associations, Dublin, December 2016.

Darley FL, Aronson AE & Brown JR. 1969, 'Clusters of deviant speech dimensions is the dysarthrias', *Journal of Speech and Hearing Disorders*, 12(3), 462–96.

Duffy JR. 2005, *Motor Speech Disorders: Substrates, differential diagnosis and management*, 2nd edn, St Louis, MO: Elsevier Mosby.

Fourcade G, Castelnovo G, Renard D & Labauge P. 2010, 'Laryngospasm as a preceding symptom of amyotrophic lateral sclerosis', *Journal of Neurology*, 257, 1929–30.

Jackson CE, McVey AL, Rudnicki S, Dimachkie MM & Barohn RJ. 2015, 'Symptom management and end-of-life care in amyotrophic lateral sclerosis', *Neurologic Clinics*, 33(4), 889–908.

Kaub-Wittemer D, von Steinbuchel N, Wasner M, Laier-Groeneveld G & Borasio GD. 2003, 'Quality of life and psychosocial issues in ventilated patient with amyotrophic lateral sclerosis and their caregivers', *Journal of Pain and Symptom Management*, 26(4), 890–6.

Kiernan MC, Vucic S, Cheah BC et al. 2011, 'Amyotrophic lateral sclerosis', *Lancet*, 377, 942–55.

King SJ, Duke MM, & O'Connor BA. 2009, 'Living with amyotrophic lateral sclerosis/motor neuron disease; decision making about "ongoing change and adaptation"', *Journal of Clinical Nursing*, 18, 745–54.

Kuhnlein P, Gdynia HJ, Sperfeld AD et al. 2008, 'Diagnosis and treatment of bulbar symptoms in amyotrophic lateral sclerosis', *Nature Clinical Practice Neurology*, 4(7), 366–74.

Ludolph A, Drory V, Hardiman O et al. 2015, 'A revision of El Escorial criteria—2015', *Amyotrophic Lateral Sclerosis and Frontotemporal Degeneration*, 16, 291–2.

Lunetta C, Lizio A, Sansone VA et al. 2016, 'Strictly monitored exercise programs reduce motor deterioration in ALS: preliminary results of a randomized controlled trial', *Journal of Neurology*, 263, 52–60.

Maslan, J, Leng X, Rees C, Blalock D & Butler S. 2011, 'Maximum phonation time in healthy older adults', *Journal of Voice*, 25(6), 709–13.

Obermann M & Lyon M 2015, 'Financial cost of amyotrophic lateral sclerosis: a case study', *Amyotrophic Lateral Sclerosis and Frontotemporal Degeneration*, 16, 54–57.

Paganoni S, Karam C, Joyce N, Bedlack R & Carter G. 2015, 'Comprehensive rehabilitative care across the spectrum of amyotrophic lateral sclerosis', *Neurorehabilitation*, 37, 53–68.

Plowman E. 2015, 'Is there a role for exercise in the management of bulbar dysfunction in amyotrophic lateral sclerosis?', *Journal of Speech, Language and Hearing Research*, 58, 1151–66.

Ringholz GM, Appel SH, Bradshaw M et al. 2005, 'Prevalence and patterns of cognitive impairment in sporadic ALS', *Neurology*, 65, 586–90.

Smith R, Pioro E, Myers K et al. 2017, 'Enhanced bulbar function in amyotrophic lateral sclerosis: the Neudexta treatment trial', *Neurotherapeutics*, 14, 762–72.

Talbot K. 2009, 'Motor neuron disease: the bare essentials', *Practical Neurology*, 9, 303–9.

Tomik B & Guiloff RJ. 2010, 'Dysarthria in amyotrophic lateral sclerosis: a review', *Amyotrophic Lateral Sclerosis*, 11, 4–15.

Traynor BJ, Alexander M, Corr B, Frost E & Hardiman O. 2003, 'Effect of a multidisciplinary amyotrophic lateral sclerosis (ALS) clinic on ALS survival: a population based study, 1996-2000', *Journal of Neurology, Neurosurgery, and Psychiatry*, 74, 1258–61.

Valdmanis PN & Rouleau GA. 2008, 'Genetics of familial amyotrophic lateral sclerosis', *Neurology*, 70, 144–x52.

Yorkston KM, Strand E, Miller R, Hillel H & Smith K. 1993, 'Speech deterioration in amyotrophic lateral sclerosis: implications for the timing of intervention', *Journal of Medical Speech–Language Pathology*, 1, 35–46.

5   Dysphagia in Parkinson's disease

Emilia Michou and Vicky Nanousi

Introduction

Dysphagia in neurodegenerative disease is a common symptom, leading to reduced quality of life and increased risk of pulmonary infections due to aspiration and unsafe swallowing. Dysphagia is a common and clinically important symptom in one of the parkinsonian syndromes, Parkinson's disease (PD), the second most frequent neurodegenerative disease (Lo & Tanner 2013).

The motor features of PD are due to degeneration of dopaminergic neurons of the substantia nigra—pars compacta. The loss of dopamine in pars compacta increases the overall inhibitory output of the basal ganglia and affects motor control. There is also increasing evidence that toxic disruption of cellular connectivity and neuronal death is formed in non-dopaminergic neurons outside the basal ganglia in PD, indicating that the pathophysiology of PD is complex.

In the hypothetical sequence of disease progression, alongside the motor system, cognitive and neurophysiological systems change (Kwan & Whitehill 2011), with patients showing reduced executive cognitive functions. Somatosensory deficits are also evident, accounting for disrupted tactile, thermal, nociception and proprioceptive sensation in PD (Conte et al. 2013). All the aforementioned provide weight to the evidence that PD is a multisystem degenerative disorder.

Dysphagia in PD is frequently characterised as 'multifaceted', given that symptoms can be observed across the continuum of deglutition although many other factors contribute to dysphagia in people with PD (PwPD). Factors associated with dysphagia in a large cohort study of 6462 PwPD included older age, longer disease duration and dementia (Cereda et al. 2014). The characteristic clinical symptoms of dysphagia in PD are shown in Suppl 5.1—Table 1. Here, we review the clinical case of a man diagnosed with idiopathic PD and dysphagia in an attempt to

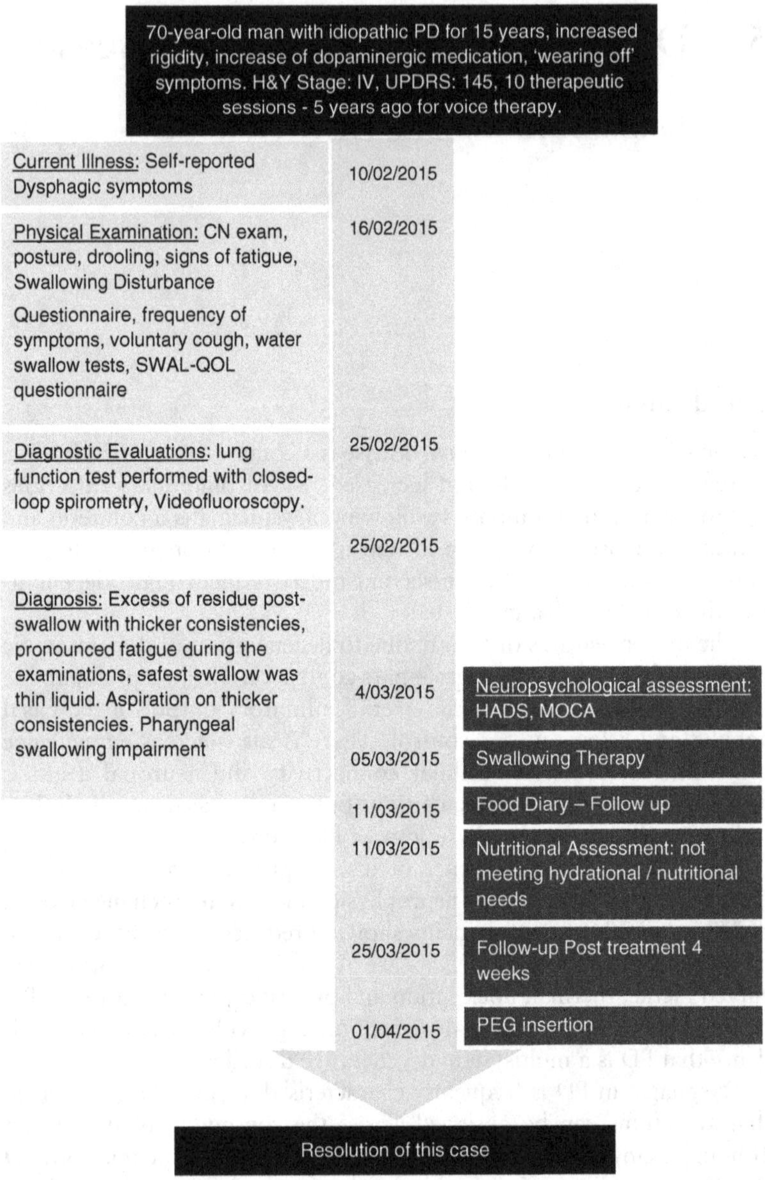

70-year-old man with idiopathic PD for 15 years, increased rigidity, increase of dopaminergic medication, 'wearing off' symptoms. H&Y Stage: IV, UPDRS: 145, 10 therapeutic sessions - 5 years ago for voice therapy.

Current Illness: Self-reported Dysphagic symptoms	10/02/2015
Physical Examination: CN exam, posture, drooling, signs of fatigue, Swallowing Disturbance	16/02/2015
Questionnaire, frequency of symptoms, voluntary cough, water swallow tests, SWAL-QOL questionnaire	
Diagnostic Evaluations: lung function test performed with closed-loop spirometry, Videofluoroscopy.	25/02/2015
	25/02/2015
Diagnosis: Excess of residue post-swallow with thicker consistencies, pronounced fatigue during the examinations, safest swallow was thin liquid. Aspiration on thicker consistencies. Pharyngeal swallowing impairment	
4/03/2015	Neuropsychological assessment: HADS, MOCA
05/03/2015	Swallowing Therapy
11/03/2015	Food Diary – Follow up
11/03/2015	Nutritional Assessment: not meeting hydrational / nutritional needs
25/03/2015	Follow-up Post treatment 4 weeks
01/04/2015	PEG insertion

Resolution of this case

Figure 5.1 Timeline according to CARE for clinical case of dysphagia in Parkinson's disease

Key: CN, cranial nerve; HADS, Hospital Anxiety and Depression Scale; H&Y, Hoehn and Yahr; MOCA, Montreal Cognitive Assessment; PD, Parkinson's disease; PEG, percutaneous gastrostomy; SWAL–QOL, swallowing quality of life; UPDRS, Unified Parkinson's Disease Rating Scale review the multidimensionality of our approach in PD with regard to the management of swallowing impairments. The CARE (CAre Report) timeline for this clinical case of dysphagia in PD is shown in Figure 5.1.

Clinical presentation

Medical and past history

Mr M. was referred to the speech and language therapy (SLT) team by the neurologist, after reported frequent choking on liquids and solids and weight loss during the last 6 months. He was a 70-year-old man diagnosed with idiopathic PD 15 years earlier. He lived with his wife, who accompanied him to the SLT clinic. The referral letter indicated that the dose of his dopaminergic medication was increased to assist Mr M. with the increased rigidity over the past months. 'Wearing-off' symptoms have also been documented. The documented neurological clinical examinations results are shown in Table 5.1. Previous clinical assessment by the SLT team took place 5 years previously, which included clinical exam, voice assessment and swallowing assessment; however, no clinical signs of unsafe swallowing were documented at the time. Nevertheless Mr M. participated in 10 sessions of voice therapy targeting voice impairments such as reduced loudness and intelligibility.

Table 5.1 Medical history and initial assessments

Medical and past history—hypothesis reasoning

Scale/Exam	Score	Information gathered
Hoehn and Yahr Scale (Hoehn & Yahr 1967)	IV	The clinical stage IV indicates that disease is 'severe but there is still ability to walk or stand unassisted'
Unified Parkinson's Disease Rating Scale (UPDRS) (Movement Disorder Society Task Force on Rating Scales for Parkinson's Disease 2003)	145	Confirmation of the disease severity. The maximum points on UPDRS are 199 (worst disability). Past scores are needed to evaluate progression. The scale is designed to examine the longitudinal progression of PD on motor and non-motor components (mood, behaviour, activities of daily living and treatment complications) (Lang et al. 2013)

(continued)

Table 5.1 (continued)

Medical and past history—hypothesis reasoning

Scale/Exam	Score	Information gathered
Disease duration	15 years	
Duration of dopaminergic medication	14 years	
Medication list at time of assessment	Rotigotine transdermal patches 4 mg, apomorphine 1 mg, levodopa 150 mg, carbidopa 37.5 mg, cardidopa/ levodopa 50/200 mg, amantadine 100 mg, clonazepam 500 mg, penicillin v potassium 10 mg, simvastatin 40 mg, Lymecycline 300 mg	Increase of dopaminergic medication show that motor symptoms are more deliberating. Dopaminergic medications producing a good effect on motor symptoms have little or no effect on symptomatic dysphagia in PD (Hunter et al. 1997, Menezes & Melo 2009, Michou et al. 2014).
Cognition and neuropsychiatric examination	Montreal Cognitive Assessment (MoCA) score: 24 Hospital Anxiety and Depression Scale (HADS): 11 in the anxiety subscale of HADS and 6 in the depression subscale	Immediate effect on the selection of the appropriate management. Dysphagia in PwPD with dementia was associated with male gender and disease duration (Cereda et al. 2014). MoCA is scoring: visuospatial, executive functions, naming, memory, attention, language, abstraction and orientation. Optimal score ≤ 25 is a cut-off point for diagnosing cognitive impairment
Voice impairment	10 therapeutic sessions—5 years previously	Dysphonia (Skodda et al. 2011) could be associated with swallowing impairments in PD (Muller et al. 2001, van Hooren et al. 2015)

Clinical hypothesis before assessment

Our initial clinical hypothesis, based on the information from the medical and past history (Table 5.1) was that Mr M. experienced signs of disease progression and that swallowing ability could be impaired, which could have coincided with the change of medication.

There is some evidence that swallowing impairments worsen with disease severity (Leopold 1996; Umemoto et al. 2011). Impaired mastication and orofacial functions are frequent in moderate–advanced PD. With regard to the medication effect on swallowing function, there is little effect on symptomatic dysphagia in PD (Hunter et al. 1997) or some effect depending on the level of degeneration (Michou et al. 2014), whereas dopaminergic medication produces a good effect on motor symptoms. Therefore, it would be important to assess the timing of presentation of symptoms and whether there are swallowing impairments during the 'on–off periods'. The 'wearing-off' symptoms are the re-emergence of parkinsonian motor symptoms, but also non-motor features such as anxiety, pain and cognitive slowing at the end of an inter-dose interval (Jankovic 2005).

Assessment

At the clinic, Mr M. showed marked instability while walking and 'freezing-of-gait' symptoms when rising from the chair in the waiting room and before entering the room. His last medication dose was received 60 minutes before the appointment, almost the time proposed as appropriate for assessment on dopaminergic medication (Michou et al. 2017). Following questions during history taking and on Mr M.'s perception on the medication change, the SLT conducted a clinical assessment: cranial nerve (CN) exam, observations of posture, drooling and signs of fatigue, as well as the Swallowing Disturbance Questionnaire (SDQ) (Manor et al. 2007), reviewing frequency of symptoms, voluntary cough as well as the Water Swallow Tests, swallowing of solid boluses and a lung function test performed with closed-loop spirometry.

Assessment of pulmonary function (Sawan et al. 2016) and cough was part of our assessment procedure given the close link of respiration and swallowing. In PwPD, in particular, respiratory impairments and other complications have been observed, including disturbances in ventilation (Gardner et al. 1986) and respiratory dysrhythmias (De Keyser & Vincken), respiratory muscle weakness (de Bruin et al. 1993), affecting both the inspiratory and the expiratory musculature. Coordination of breathing and swallowing is impaired in PwPD (Gross et al. 2008), with PwPD showing significantly more post-swallow inhalation.

The SLT department has already established a close working relationship with the neuropsychologists, who had already assessed Mr M.'s cognition. The neuropsychologist administered the Montreal Cognitive Assessment (Nasreddine et al. 2005), and the Hospital Anxiety and Depression Scale (Zigmond & Snaith 1983). Mr M. showed marked 'feelings of anxiety'. At the end of the session, Mr M. was asked to complete the SWAL–QOL questionnaire (McHorney et al. 2002).

Findings from initial assessment

Mr M. informed us that his swallowing ability changed and he had problems with tongue control, frequent coughing and noticeable drooling. He felt that 'there is something left after the swallow' (pointing towards the upper part of the larynx). He avoided food and liquid consumption during 'wearing-off' periods but he did not face any major difficulty with the tablets (consumed with some puree consistency food). It was more difficult for him to use liquid for his medication, mainly because of difficulty propelling the tablet backwards. Fatigue was a major issue, with swallowing becoming more difficult towards the end of the day.

The results from the CN examination demonstrated reduced jaw lateralisation, and weak jaw opening against resistance (pathological findings for CN V), whereas lingual protrusion and lateralisation showed marked weakness (pathological findings for CN XII). General sensation in the oral cavity was adequate but reduced taste sensation on sour and bitter stimuli was evident on the posterior third of the tongue (CN IX). The water swallow tests indicated that there is an overall decreased swallowing speed, reduced laryngeal elevation and reflexive coughing in larger quantities. Mr M.'s voluntary cough after water swallowing was deemed adequate; nonetheless, he showed overt signs of unsafe swallowing and aspiration.

From his answers to the SDQ, the questions covering impairments of pharyngeal phase of the swallow were scored 'with higher frequency' (Suppl 5.1). The raw scores of Mr M. 's answers to SWAL-QOL are shown in the Suppl 5.2.

Based on these results, it was decided that his swallowing function should be reviewed with formal imaging assessment using videofluoroscopic swallowing study (VFSS).

Formal imaging of swallowing

Clips of swallowing examination (puree [40% w/v EZ-Paque], liquid [60% w/v] and saliva swallowing) are shown in Suppl 5.3–5.5. Mr M. was assessed when 'on' medication, 90 minutes after the last dose. The major impairment on VFSS was aspiration at but not below the vocal folds, with reflexive coughing, and Mr M. showed fatigue and inability to complete manoeuvres. For the thicker consistencies, there was marked residue in the valleculae and the pyriform sinuses post-swallow. Reflexive coughing was observed after swallowing of pudding-like consistency. The worst Penetration/Aspiration score (Rosenbek et al. 1996) was 5 on pudding (Suppl 5.3). Interestingly, the patient requested the termination of the examination, before the therapist could trial different boluses (solids and carbonated liquids), as well as the anterior–posterior view. The patient showed signs of fatigue and breathlessness that subsided 5 minutes later. The median oral transit time for thicker boluses was longer compared with that for thin fluids (1.62 s vs 1.36 s), similar to the pharyngeal swallow delay (median 0.61 s vs 0.14 s, respectively). The swallows when aspiration was evident had longer pharyngeal transit time compared with the non-aspirative swallows, whereas airway closure duration did not show any change. Aspiration occurred post-swallow, with residue in the pyriform sinuses being the source of material misdirected to the trachea.

Assessments summary

Both the respiratory and swallowing system showed impairments and corroborated Mr M.'s perception of his swallowing ability. The findings of interest were the excess residue post-swallow with thicker consistencies and the pronounced fatigue during the examinations. The pharyngeal swallowing impairment (increased pharyngeal transit time with adequate airway closure) was indicative of the advanced dysphagia stage in PwPD (see Table 5.1). One of the symptoms usually observed is incomplete cricopharyngeal sphincter relaxation, which can indicate either hypertonic sphincter or result from the reduced forward and upward movement of the hyolaryngeal complex, and even from weak propulsion forces and pharyngeal peristalsis. Sensory loss of receptors at the level of the tongue base could also account for increased residue in the vallecular spaces. Mr M.'s hydration and nutritional status are affected by the swallowing impairments and the progressive nature of the disease will further affect his pulmonary function as well as his swallowing.

Management

In order to keep hydration levels stable, Mr M. was asked to continue swallowing small sips of water regularly during the day. He was referred to the 'nutrition team' for further assessment. Given the close link of dysphagia to nutritional status, it was imperative to examine his nutritional status. A systematic review found that 3–60% of patients with PD were at risk of malnutrition (Sheard et al. 2013). Progressive weight loss, and especially fat mass loss (Markus et al. 1993), is a major feature in PD starting 2–4 years before diagnosis (Chen et al. 2003).

Following discussions with Mr M., a decision was made that he would continue eating more moist consistencies to compensate for the difficulties in the pharyngeal stage of swallowing. A food diary was also initiated with information on the consistency of the food, the meals frequency, and any signs of impaired swallow or excessive fatigue during completing meals throughout the day.

While the team waited for the complete assessment by the nutrition team, a second referral was instigated to the respiratory physiotherapy team.

Even though his clinical profile showed signs of deterioration and advanced dysphagia, therapy was initiated. A week later, his food diary showed his preference for softer consistencies and coughing was frequent during mealtime. A fibreoptic endoscopic evaluation of swallowing (FEES) took place to verify safety for the nectar-like or thinner consistencies, and showed marked residue in the pyriform sinuses which were reduced with a liquid clearing swallow.

Mr M. underwent therapy for 2 weeks in the clinic (3 days/week) and was reviewed again 4 weeks post-initial assessment. For the first part of the sessions, the speech and language therapist was trialling alternate boluses of two different consistencies deemed as safer (liquid and puree boluses) with different tastes, given that there is evidence of bolus supplementation with piperine speeding the swallow response and improving swallow safety (Rofes et al. 2014). When signs of fatigue were evident, the patient was asked to stop and rest. During the sessions, Mr M. also underwent biofeedback while he was being scoped. There is evidence that biofeedback with the use of videos of normal swallowing process, videos obtained with FEES showing the individual's swallowing impairments, and the effects of compensatory techniques in a paradigm called video-assisted swallowing therapy, could reduce the post-swallow residue in PwPD (Manor et al. 2013). However, Mr M.'s attention level was not adequate and he could not understand the view of his FEES and how to organise swallows while reducing the amount of residue. After this, the patient completed the swallowing reaction time task (Michou et al. 2012), utilising pharyngeal manometry with a solid-state manometric catheter. In this task, the patient was required to complete normally paced swallows and fast-paced swallows, as well as swallows within a pre-conditioned time window shown on the desktop with a single line. Recordings were collected via the manometric pressure transducer and, if the pharyngeal pressure collected via the transducer reached above a predetermined threshold, a swallow was registered. Mr M. had to swallow within the pre-conditioned time window for his swallow to be 'successful'. Mr M. expressed that for him less visual information and fewer instructions to follow was less taxing and confusing. Ten swallows were trialled during each session, taking into consideration any signs of fatigue.

Outcome

The SWAL–QOL was repeated again at weeks 2 and 4 after the initial assessments to observe changes after the subsequent management (see Suppl 5.2) to monitor therapy outcome. There were clear signs of improvement of the overall patient's quality of life (QoL) and a reduction in the 'symptoms' overall subscale. However, a progressive motor and peripheral pulmonary impairment was noted following further examinations by the physiotherapy team. The food diary that Mr M. kept was discussed with the nutrition team and was compared with their nutritional assessment. The multidisciplinary team (MDT) was informed of all the results and concluded that his total daily intake was not sufficient to cover his nutritional and hydration needs. It was therefore proposed that an alternative feeding route would be of benefit, while Mr M. would continue oral intake of liquids and puree consistency until further assessment. Mr M. was then reviewed by the nutrition team on a regular basis at his home setting, and he attended swallow clinics every two months, until he was unable to travel due to his balance problems. Six months after the percutaneous endoscopic gastrostomy (PEG) insertion, his parkinsonian motor symptoms deteriorated and he died after an accidental fall.

Reflection and clinical messages

Dysphagia in PD can result in impaired safety, aspiration pneumonia, malnutrition and dehydration, and consequently to a well-documented decline of QoL. The underlying neurodegenerative mechanisms in the central and peripheral nervous systems affect not only the oral propulsion of the bolus, but also the propagation of the bolus through the pharyngeal stage towards the oesophagus.

Given the neurodegenerative nature of the disease, the clinician assessing and managing PwPD must be adept at recognising not only the clinical signs of dysphagia but also the underlying pathophysiology, the evolution and the variation of symptomatology with disease progression. It is important to state that there is no evidence that the changes in swallowing function follow a progressive pattern. On the contrary, what is evident is that each patient shows a distinct progression pattern.

From a clinical perspective, disease duration and the frequency of swallowing problems, which could be higher in the later stages, may account for the clinically significant dysphagia problems in PD. Indeed, there is insufficient information about the appropriate time of initial swallowing assessment and usually patients receive therapy when swallowing function is deteriorating in the more severe and advanced disease stages.

Although new treatments have been proposed, including oromotor exercises (Argolo et al. 2013), electrical stimulation (Heijnen et al. 2012; Baijens et al. 2013) and expiratory muscle strength training (Pitts et al. 2009; Troche et al. 2010), there is missing evidence about which patients and what type of swallowing impairments can be targeted using these therapeutic approaches. Understanding the patient's ability and the effect of neurodegeneration on other systems, such as fatigue, cognition, pain and respiration, are key components during the clinical decision-making with regard to therapy duration, therapy intensity as well as the choice of therapeutic approach. It could be argued that therapeutic techniques for PwPD and dysphagia should be providing input to more than one function, i.e. cognition, taste, proprioception, attention, muscle training and respiratory training, because dysphagia in this population in multifaceted.

To conclude, the key points to be raised in this case study are that there are marked differences in presentation of swallowing impairments among PwPD; not all patients will experience all symptoms and not at the same period of disease progression. The above also indicate that the clinical assessment needs to be thorough.

References

Argolo N, Sampaio M, Pihno P, Melo A & Nobrega A. 2013. 'Do swallowing exercises improve swallowing dynamic and quality of life in Parkinson's disease?' *NeuroRehabilitation*, 32, 949–55.

Baijens LW, Speyer R, Passos VL et al. 2013. 'Surface electrical stimulation in dysphagic Parkinson patients: a randomized clinical trial', *Laryngoscope*, 123, E38–44.

Cereda E, Cilia R, Klersy C et al. 2014, 'Swallowing disturbances in Parkinson's disease: a multivariate analysis of contributing factors', *Parkinsonism Related Disorders*, 20, 1382–7.

Chen H, Zhang SM, Hernan MA, Willett WC & Ascherio A. 2003. 'Weight loss in Parkinson's disease', *Annals of Neurology*, 53, 676–9.

Conte A, Khan N, Defazio G, Rothwell JC & Berardelli A. 2013, 'Pathophysiology of somatosensory abnormalities in Parkinson disease', *Nature Reviews Neurology*, 9, 687–97.

de Bruin PF, De Bruin VM, Lees AJ & Pride NB. 1993, 'Effects of treatment on airway dynamics and respiratory muscle strength in Parkinson's disease. *American Review Respiratory Disorders*, 148, 1576–80.

De Keyser J & Vincken W, 1985. 'L-Dopa-induced respiratory disturbance in Parkinson's disease suppressed by tiapride', *Neurology*, 35, 235–7.

Gardner WN, Meah MS & Bass C. 1986. Controlled study of respiratory responses during prolonged measurement in patients with chronic hyperventilation', *Lancet*, 2, 826–30.

Gross RD. Atwood CW, Ross SB, Eichhorn KA, Olszewski JW & Doyle PJ. 2008. 'The coordination of breathing and swallowing in Parkinson's disease', *Dysphagia*, 23, 136–45.

Heijnen BJ, Speyer R, Baijens LW & Bogaardt HC. 2012 'Neuromuscular electrical stimulation versus traditional therapy in patients with Parkinson's disease and oropharyngeal dysphagia: effects on quality of life', *Dysphagia*, 27, 336–45.

Hoehn MM & Yahr MD. 1967, 'Parkinsonism: onset, progression and mortality', *Neurology*, 17, 427–42.

Hunter PC, Crameri J, Austin S, Woodward MC & Hughes AJ. 1997, 'Response of parkinsonian swallowing dysfunction to dopaminergic stimulation', *Journal of Neurology Neurosurgery and Psychiatry*, 63, 579–83.

Jankovic J. 2005, 'Motor fluctuations and dyskinesias in Parkinson's disease: clinical manifestations', *Movement Disorders*, 20(Suppl. 11), S11–16.

Kwan LC & Whitehill TL. 2011, 'Perception of speech by individuals with Parkinson's disease: a review', *Parkinsons Disease*, article ID 389767, 1–11.

Lang AE, Eberly S, Goetz CG et al. & LABS-PD Investigators 2013, 'Movement disorder society unified Parkinson disease rating scale experiences in daily living: longitudinal changes and correlation with other assessments', *Movement Disorders*, 28, 1980–6.

Leopold NA. 1996, 'A comment on quantitative assessment of oral and pharyngeal function in Parkinson's disease', *Dysphagia*, 11, 274–5.

Lo R & Tanner C. 2013, 'Epidemiology', in: Pahwa R. & Lyons, K. (eds), *Handbook of Parkinson's Disease*, 5th edn, Boca Raton, FL: CRC Press.

McHorney CA, Robbins J, Lomax K et al. 2002, 'The SWAL-QOL and SWAL-CARE outcomes tool for oropharyngeal dysphagia in adults: III. Documentation of reliability and validity', *Dysphagia*, 17, 97–114.

Manor Y, Giladi N, Cohen A, Fliss DM & Cohen JT. 2007, 'Validation of a swallowing disturbance questionnaire for detecting dysphagia in patients with Parkinson's disease', *Movement Disorders*, 22, 1917–21.

Manor Y, Mootanah R, Freud D, Giladi N & Cohen JT. 2013, 'Video-assisted swallowing therapy for patients with Parkinson's disease', *Parkinsonism Related Disorders*, 19, 207–11.

Markus HS, Tomkins AM & Stern GM. 1993, 'Increased prevalence of under-nutrition in Parkinson's disease and its relationship to clinical disease parameters', *Journal of Neural Transmission Parkinson's Disease Dementia Section*, 5, 117–25.

Menezes C & Melo A. 2009, 'Does levodopa improve swallowing dysfunction in Parkinson's disease patients?' *Journal of Clinical Pharmacy and Therapeutics*, 34, 673–6.

Michou E, Mastan A, Ahmed S, Mistry S & Hamdy S. 2012, 'Examining the role of carbonation and temperature on water swallowing performance: a swallowing reaction-time study', *Chemical Senses*, 37, 799–807.

Michou E, Hamdy S, Harris M et al. 2014, 'Characterization of corticobulbar pharyngeal neurophysiology in dysphagic patients with Parkinson's disease', *Clinical Gastroenterology and Hepatology*, 12, 2037–45, e1–4.

Michou E, Kobylecki C & Hamdy S. 2017, 'Dysphagia in Parkinson's disease,' in: Ekberg O (ed.), *Dysphagia*, Berlin, Heidelberg: Springer.

Movement Disorder Society Task Force on Rating Scales for Parkinson's Disease. 2003, 'The Unified Parkinson's Disease Rating Scale (UPDRS): status and recommendations', *Movement Disorders*, 18, 738–50.

Muller J, Wenning GK, Verny M et al. 2001, 'Progression of dysarthria and dysphagia in postmortem-confirmed parkinsonian disorders', *Archives of Neurology*, 58, 259–64.

Nasreddine ZS, Phillips NA, Bedirian V et al. 2005, 'The Montreal Cognitive Assessment, MoCA: a brief screening tool for mild cognitive impairment' *Journal of American Geriatric Society*, 53, 695–99.

Pitts T, Bolser D, Rosenbek J, Troche M, Okun MS & Sapienza C. 2009, 'Impact of expiratory muscle strength training on voluntary cough and swallow function in Parkinson disease', *Chest*, 135, 1301–8.

Rofes L, Arreola V, Martin A & Clave P. 2014, 'Effect of oral piperine on the swallow response of patients with oropharyngeal dysphagia', *Journal of Gastroenterology*, 49, 1517–23.

Rosenbek JC, Robbins JA, Roecker EB, Coyle JL & Wood JL. 1996, 'A penetration-aspiration scale', *Dysphagia*, 11, 93–8.

Sawan T, Harris ML, Kobylecki C, Baijens L, Van Hooren M & Michou E. 2016. 'Lung function testing on and off dopaminergic medication in Parkinson's disease patients with and without dysphagia', *Movement Disorders Clinical Practice*, 3, 146–150.

Sheard JM, Ash S, Mellick GD, Silburn PA & Kerr GK. 2013, 'Markers of disease severity are associated with malnutrition in Parkinson's disease', *PLoS One*, 8, no. e57986.

Skodda S, Flasskamp A & Schlegel U. 2011, 'Instability of syllable repetition in Parkinson's disease—influence of levodopa and deep brain stimulation', *Movement Disorders*, 26, 728–30.

Troche MS, Okun MS, Rosenbek JC et al. 2010, 'Aspiration and swallowing in Parkinson disease and rehabilitation with EMST: a randomized trial', *Neurology*, 75, 1912–19.

Umemoto G, Tsuboi Y, Kitashima A, Furuya H & Kikuta T. 2011, 'Impaired food transportation in Parkinson's disease related to lingual bradykinesia', *Dysphagia*, 26, 250–5.

Van Hooren MR, Baijens LW, Vos R et al. 2015, 'Voice- and swallow-related quality of life in idiopathic Parkinson's disease', *Laryngoscope*, 126(2), 408–14.

Zigmond AS & Snaith RP. 1983, 'The Hospital Anxiety and Depression Scale', *Acta Psychiatrica Scandinavica*, 67, 361–70.

6 Dysphagia associated with head and neck cancer

Grainne Brady and Justin Roe

Introduction

This clinical case considers the complexities of management of dysphagia following treatment for head and neck cancer (HNC). In this chapter, we consider the side effects of radical treatments, including surgery and chemoradiotherapy (CRT), on the patient's swallowing function and the management options available to clinicians. The chapter includes the perspective of a person coping with dysphagia after radical surgery and adjuvant CRT for HNC. This case also illustrates the complexity when multiple services are accessed.

Presenting concerns

A 73-year-old man was referred to a specialist head and neck speech and language therapy service with dysphagia on a background history of T2N2b squamous cell carcinoma (SCC) of the right base of the tongue. Previous medical history also includes type 1 diabetes and cardiac issues. He was previously treated with surgical excision, including partial laser glossectomy, and a right modified neck dissection including lymph nodes levels I–IV, with postoperative CRT. He was referred for speech and language therapy at a tertiary referral centre for assessment five years after completing his radical HNC treatment. Referral information included a history of four episodes of aspiration pneumonia over a 24-month period.

Clinical findings

The patient's initial diagnosis of T2N2b SCC of the right base of tongue was made in the USA and was treated with surgery and post-operative CRT at an independent hospital in the UK. A prophylactic gastrostomy tube was placed before the CRT. However, this was removed shortly after treatment when he resumed oral intake.

Although previously seen by a speech and language therapist (SLT) following surgery and CRT, the patient did not recall receiving any specific rehabilitation interventions. He underwent two videofluoroscopic examinations in 2009 and 2012. From reports accessed from the assessing centres, it was documented that he presented overt aspiration on thin and thick liquids. He was previously recommended thickened fluids and a supraglottic swallow. Information was very limited with regard to the nature and extent of his oropharyngeal dysphagia. Although surgical follow-up continued in the USA with a head and neck surgeon, regular follow-up also continued with a radiation oncologist in the UK.

The patient complained of persistent coughing while eating and drinking, and was very concerned about recent repeated episodes of pneumonia. As a very active man enjoying a number of sporting and social activities, he found coughing during mealtimes and periods of illness due to pneumonia were having a significant impact on his quality of life (QoL). He was very anxious to find both a cause and a solution for his swallowing difficulty.

On oromotor assessment a right-sided marginal mandibular weakness and reduced jaw opening were noted. Diet was restricted, avoiding many meat consistencies due to difficulties chewing and swallowing. Despite coughing on fluids, and previous recommendations, intake of thin fluids continued and he expressed finding thickened fluids unacceptable.

Surgery and/or CRT is the mainstay treatment for HNC. One of the most common and profound effects of HNC and its treatment are the acute and long-term difficulties with eating and drinking (Paleri et al., 2013). Swallowing function has been identified as a key priority for patients with HNC, not only at the point of diagnosis and during CRT, but also up to 1 year after completion (Patterson et al., 2014; Roe et al., 2014).

Surgical treatment results in tissue loss with subsequent changes to the anatomy and structural relationships. Swallowing difficulties can change over time with greater prevalence of oedema in the acute postoperative phase followed by atrophy and scarring in the longer term (Patterson et al., 2016). Surgery can also result in nerve damage, causing both motor and sensory deficits. Dysphagia severity depends on a number of factors including baseline functioning, extent of resection and type of reconstruction (Lam & Samman, 2013). Adjuvant CRT is likely to have a further detrimental effect on swallowing function (Patterson et al., 2016).

Based on the clinical presentation and previous instrumental examinations, this patient presented with radiologically confirmed aspiration. It is most likely that this long-standing swallowing difficulty was a result of his previous curative treatment, which involved both surgery and CRT. However, given the new onset of chest sepsis and increased difficulties reported by the patient, it was hypothesized that any pre-existing dysphagia was complicated by late radiation-associated dysphagia (RAD) (Hutcheson et al., 2012). Respiratory decompensation secondary to chronic aspiration, as confirmed by videofluoroscopy, was also considered to be a contributory factor (Bianchi & Cantarella, 2011).

Late RAD is defined as the occurrence of swallowing difficulties after a long interval of functional swallowing—often five years or more (Hutcheson et al., 2015). The condition is often characterised by impaired hyolaryngeal excursion, pharyngeal constriction and tongue-base retraction causing pharyngeal residue and aspiration (Hutcheson et al., 2012). The underlying pathophysiology for such impairments may involve severe fibrosis, muscle atrophy and cranial neuropathies (Hutcheson et al., 2017a, 2017b).

There is an increasing body of evidence with regard to preventative strategies to reduce the risk and severity of dysphagia following HNC treatment, which can be introduced before, during and after CRT, including the maintenance of eating and drinking, the selective use of feeding tubes and prophylactic swallowing exercises (Paleri et al., 2014). Patients are generally encouraged to eat and drink during their radiotherapy. Prolonged periods of nil by mouth are associated with poorer swallowing outcomes due to deconditioning and atrophy of the swallowing musculature (Paleri et al., 2014).

There has been much debate in the literature about the use of tube feeding during CRT. Although some advocate the use of prophylactic gastrostomy placement before treatment in the presence of functional swallowing, others take a more reactive approach, placing a nasogastric feeding tube when the patient is no longer able to maintain sufficient oral nutrition and hydration. It has been hypothesized that patients with prophylactic gastrostomy may avoid eating and drinking earlier, leading to increased periods of nil by mouth status (Patterson et al., 2016). Studies have shown that as many as 30–50% of patients are able to maintain sufficient nutrition and hydration without augmentation with tube feeding during their radiotherapy (Clavel et al., 2011; Bhayani et al., 2013; Roe et al., 2014). However, others argue that prophylactic gastrostomy tubes are required to ensure fewer hospital admissions or breaks in treatment (Shaw et al., 2015). A recent randomized controlled trial has found no impact of prophylactic tubes on weight loss during treatment (Brown et al., 2017). Others have reported that a nasogastric tube may act as a pharyngeal stent, as fewer patients fed by this method seem to develop upper oesophageal stricture requiring dilatation (Paleri et al., 2014).

The introduction of swallowing exercises prophylactically to optimize swallowing has been investigated in a number of studies (Kraaijenga et al., 2014; Paleri et al., 2014; Peng et al., 2015; Virani et al., 2015). This patient had a prophylactic gastrostomy tube placed before his CRT and he was reliant on this tube for a period during and after his CRT. He recalls being 'unable to swallow' for a period; however, no detail was provided about the duration of nil by mouth status. The patient does not recall a baseline pre-treatment assessment with a SLT or being provided with prophylactic swallowing exercise regimens. The lack of baseline assessment data, coupled with the absence of prophylactic exercises, is a potential risk factor for increased severity of long-term swallowing difficulties.

Although much of the literature in HNC is focused on the prevention of dysphagia after treatment, up to 60% of patients do experience dysphagia after treatment (Shune et al., 2012). It is clear that, based on the clinical presentation, this patient experienced dysphagia after treatment. The extent to which dysphagia before treatment may have been a contributing factor is not clear due to the absence of baseline swallowing measures. The benefits of swallowing therapy for dysphagia after treatment completion are clinically evident and, as such, rehabilitative therapy post treatment is widely supported by the multidisciplinary team (Virani et al., 2015). Although this man did have a radiologically confirmed swallowing impairment after treatment, he does not recall receiving rehabilitative exercises following his videofluoroscopic examinations. In addition, there is limited detail in the acquired reports, with recommendations being made in the absence of details of the nature and extent of his oropharyngeal dysphagia.

Table 6.1 Clinical care timeline

November 2008	T2N2bM0 SCC tongue base diagnosed in the USA
December 2008	Right base of tongue laser partial glossectomy with modified right neck dissection—independent hospital in the UK. Prophylactic PEG pre-CRT
February 2009	Completed postoperative CRT—independent hospital in the UK. PEG removed post-treatment

(continued)

Table 6.1 (continued)

July 2009	Initial SLT assessment, videofluoroscopy. Recommendations: thickened fluids—independent hospital in the UK
Jan 2013	Re-referral to SLT. Videofluoroscopy, silent aspiration, supraglottic swallow—private hospital in the UK
July 2014	Re-referral to SLT at a head and neck specialist service; 24-history of repeated pneumonia
August 2014	Videofluoroscopy to guide dysphagia therapy
September 2014	Repeat videofluoroscopy as outcome measure
October 2014	SLT input in USA—neuromuscular electrical stimulation (NMES) as adjunct to swallow therapy
December 2014	Repeated chest infections
January 2015	SLT review—specialist head and neck centre—safe swallowing guidelines, oral care and resume standard dysphagia therapy exercises
February 2015	SLT input in USA—NMES
September 2015	SLT review—specialist head and neck centre—safe swallowing guidelines, oral care and resume standard dysphagia therapy exercises. Aim to review in 12 months
July 2016	Further repeated chest infections.
August 2016	SLT review- Specialist head and neck centre-videofluoroscopy- compensatory strategy- FEES as biofeedback for effective use of compensatory strategies
September 2016	Elective admission for cardiac surgery postponed due to chest infection
December 2016	Fall with cervical spine fracture—conservative management with neck brace
February 2017	Cardiac surgery —complicated postoperative course with complete heart block and emergency pacemaker
May 2017	SLT review—specialist head and neck centre—FEES—compensatory strategies—EMST
June 2017	Returned to USA—due for repeat FEES as outcome measure and ongoing close follow-up on return to UK

Diagnostic focus and assessment

Clinical evaluation of swallowing was completed on referral to the speech and language therapy service five years after treatment:

Clinical assessment of swallowing

The patient complained of persistent coughing while eating and drinking and was very concerned about recent repeated episodes of pneumonia. He presented with a history of four chest infections over the past two years, one of which required a prolonged inpatient hospital stay. He recalls swallowing difficulties during his CRT, during which he was reliant on a gastrostomy tube. He reports making a good post-treatment recovery, returning to a near-normal diet. He reported some persisting xerostomia. Oro-motor assessment indicated the following:

- Right-sided marginal mandibular weakness;
- Mildly reduced jaw opening;
- Intact strength, speed and range of motion of the tongue;
- Symmetrical elevation of the soft palate on phonation;
- Voluntary cough achieved.

Swallowing was assessed on thin fluids (water). Swallowing initiation was present with hyolaryngeal movement present on palpation. Delayed and significant coughing was noted post-swallowing, indicative of potential aspiration. For this reason, the 100-ml water swallow test (Patterson et al., 2011), which is part of our standard assessment protocol, was not administered.

Based on clinical assessment it would appear that the patient had been experiencing radiologically confirmed aspiration for some time.

Table 6.2 Outcome measures in head and neck cancer

Measure/time point	Baseline
PSS-HN normalcy of diet	70 (avoids meats)
PSS-HN eating in public	100 (no restrictions)
PSS-HN understandability of speech	100 (fully intelligible)
MIO	33mm
MDADI global score	4
GRBAS Grade	0

MDADI, MD Anderson Dysphagia Inventory (Chen et al., 2001); MIO, Maximum Interincisor Opening; GRBAS Perceptual Voice Evaluation (Hirano, 1981); PSS-HN, Performance Status Scale for Head and Neck Cancer (List et al., 1990).

More recently, however, it appeared that aspiration was now leading to repeated chest infections. Further objective assessment of swallowing using videofluoroscopy was recommended to ascertain if the patient's swallowing difficulties related to the late effects of previous radical treatment undertaken 5 years previously, or resulted from the original functional impairment after treatment. It was hypothesized that this diagnosis could be confirmed, based on comparison of images and reports from the previous examinations completed in 2009 and 2012.

Instrumental evaluation

A videofluoroscopy was undertaken after clinical assessment. This demonstrated a pharyngeal dysphagia characterized by the following:

- Collection of residue noted at the valleculae secondary to reduced tongue base retraction and only partial epiglottic movement;
- Incomplete anterior hyoid excursion with reduced pharyngo-oesophageal segment opening. Subsequent partial obstruction of the bolus flow with collection of residue at the pyriform sinus;
- Incomplete laryngeal vestibular closure with penetration during the swallow across consistencies;
- Silent aspiration across consistencies post-swallow due to uncleared penetrated material;
- An effortful swallow observed to reduce the volume of residue and a clearing cough post-swallow observed to reduce but not eliminate the volume of aspiration/penetration.

On previous examinations, aspiration of thin and thickened fluids was noted; however, silent aspiration was not reported. Previous external reports did not document any findings in relation to swallowing diet options and there was little to no information about swallowing pathophysiology.

Deterioration in swallowing function was confirmed with reduced sensation, resulting in silent aspiration. A diagnosis of late RAD on a background of a probable persisting impairment in swallow function after radical treatment for HNC was made.

Therapeutic focus and assessment

Intervention 1

The assessment findings and images from the recent videofluoroscopy were discussed with the patient. Significant time was spent explaining the mechanism by which surgery followed by radiotherapy can affect swallowing. A management plan was implemented which included advice on oral hygiene, safe swallowing recommendations, compensatory techniques and rehabilitative exercises.

Oral hygiene

Given the known risk of aspiration pneumonia with poor oral hygiene (Langmore et al., 1998) the importance of optimizing mouth care was explained to the patient.

Safe swallowing recommendations

Given the known risk of aspiration, the patient was advised to sit upright for all oral intake and to remain upright and mobile for a short period after his meals. Based on videofluoroscopy findings, the patient was advised to take small sips of thin fluids to help reduce the volume of aspiration.

Compensatory techniques

In the setting of late RAD, compensatory techniques have been found to be clinically effective (Hutcheson et al., 2012). The effortful swallow that is designed to improve tongue-base movement posteriorly and thus improve clearance from the valleculae was introduced following videofluoroscopy (Logemann, 1998).

Rehabilitative exercises:

- To address anterior hyoid movement the Shaker exercise (Shaker et al., 1997) was introduced;
- To address tongue base to posterior pharyngeal wall approximation, the Masako (Fujiu & Logemann, 1996) was introduced.

Rehabilitation prescription was as follows:

- Shaker: sustained head lift (60 seconds) and repeated head lifts (30 repetitions) completed 3 times, 3 times daily;
- Masako: (tongue hold technique) 5–10 repetitions, completed 3 times daily.

It has been highlighted in the literature that the tongue-hold technique should be introduced in conjunction with the Shaker, to compensate for reduced anterior hyoid movement (Doeltgen et al., 2009). A self-directed dysphagia home therapy programme was advised, because the patient had to travel a number of hours to attend appointments at the tertiary referral centre where he wanted to receive his care. Email and telephone contact was maintained to provide support to and receive feedback from the patient.

Outcome measurement

After eight weeks of self-directed dysphagia therapy, a repeat videofluoroscopy was completed to measure any change in swallowing physiology following dysphagia rehabilitation. No change in swallowing was noted with comparable findings to the initial examination. The patient had, however, remained well with no further episodes of chest infection. He reported being extremely diligent with regard to his oral hygiene and remained very active, playing golf regularly. He reported an improvement in his swallowing function, found the effortful swallow technique useful and felt more comfortable while eating and drinking. He reported that he found the exercises were helping and he was disappointed to hear that the objective assessment results remained unchanged. The Performance Status Scale for Head and Neck Cancer (PSS-HN; List et al., 1990) diet score also remained unchanged. It has been reported that swallowing impairments, which are refractory to traditional intervention techniques, are consistent with a diagnosis of late RAD (Hutcheson, 2012). The patient was advised to continue with the previous management plan, including safe swallowing guidelines, oral hygiene and compensatory techniques. He also chose to continue with rehabilitative exercises because he felt that they continued to benefit him.

Intervention 2

Three months later the patient was in the UK and requested a review just before returning to the USA. He remained well with no signs of aspiration. He continued with his dysphagia management programme, including safe eating guidelines, oral hygiene, compensatory strategies and dysphagia rehabilitation exercises. He reported that he was doing his exercises with less frequency but still continuing with the exercise regimen on a regular basis. The patient reported that he felt the swallowing interventions were helpful. Outcome measure scores remained unchanged from the initial meeting.

Intervention 3

The patient requested a further review almost a year later when he returned to the UK after a trip to the USA. While in the USA he was seen for review by the head and neck surgeon who originally diagnosed his cancer. He was referred to a speech and language pathologist for intervention. He underwent a weeklong course of NMES therapy and given an extensive, ongoing, home programme of oromotor and swallowing exercises to complete three times daily. The patient reported feeling overwhelmed by the self-directed exercise programme, which was taking on average an hour to complete. He recently had another chest infection and was still recovering from this at the time of review. He did not recall having a baseline instrumental evaluation of swallowing prior before commencing the course of NMES and home rehabilitation programme. The patient had previously been advised that NMES intervention is not widely used in the UK because the evidence base for this intervention remained limited. In addition there was a lack of high-quality controlled trials reported in systematic reviews, particularly in the treatment of head and neck radiation-related swallowing impairment. It was explained that, at that time, NMES was not in use outside of clinical trials in the NHS pending a review by the National Institute for Health and Care Excellence (NICE).

Outcome measurement

A repeat videofluoroscopy was completed to understand the nature and extent of his dysphagia after his recent interventions. This demonstrated a pharyngeal dysphagia characterized by the following:

- Vallecular residue due to reduced tongue base retraction and incomplete epiglottic inversion;
- Reduced hyolaryngeal excursion with penetration observed during the swallow across consistencies;
- Subsequent silent aspiration of penetrated material across consistencies post-swallow;
- Pharyngo-oesophageal segment opening appeared improved with free passage of the bolus and subsequent reduced residue post-swallow compared with previous examination;
- An effortful swallow was no longer effective, resulting in increased volume of aspiration across consistencies.

The repeat examination showed a biomechanical change in swallowing function and a compensatory strategy that had previously improved swallowing safety and efficiency was no longer effective and now resulted in increased volume of aspiration. In a randomized trial of patients receiving NMES with traditional swallowing rehabilitation exercises versus sham NMES with traditional swallowing rehabilitation exercises, NMES did not augment the benefit of swallowing exercise and the latter were not effective on their own either (Langmore et al., 2016). Given the observed airway closure difficulties on videofluoroscopy, a fibreoptic endoscopic evaluation of swallowing (FEES) was completed immediately afterwards, as a bio-feedback method to instruct the patient on how to successfully complete the supraglottic swallow as a compensatory technique. This was critical, because a previous study has shown that 57.7% of patients are unable to achieve voluntary airway closure when evaluated with nasendoscopy (Hirst et al., 1998). It was interesting that, despite undergoing explanations of videofluoroscopic studies previously, this patient found FEES to be highly valuable in developing his understanding of his swallowing.

The dysphagia management plan was revised to include the compensatory technique of the supraglottic swallow in addition to the safe swallow guidelines, oral hygiene advice and rehabilitative swallowing (Shaker and Masako) exercises as before.

The patient reported that he was due for admission for elective cardiac thoracic surgery for an aortic valve replacement. Given the known history of silent aspiration, careful attention was paid to provide full and detailed handover to the speech and language therapy team at the cardiothoracic centre to ensure that the patient could be closely monitored during his postoperative recovery. The cardiac surgery was postponed in the first instance due to a further episode of pneumonia, and then due to a fall, which resulted in a fracture of the cervical spine. The spinal injury was managed at his local general hospital so, again, due diligence was required to provide accurate reports about swallowing status to the managing medical and speech and language therapy team. The patient was seen by the speech and language therapy team at the local hospital where thickened fluids were recommended in the absence of instrumental evaluation. This differing approach to dysphagia management may reflect the lack of experience of the local speech and language therapy team in managing HNC caseloads. Due to the cervical spine fracture, the patient required a neck brace for a number of months and he felt that the reduced mobility resulted in deterioration in swallowing function. All dysphagia rehabilitation exercises were discontinued. The cardiac surgery was undertaken almost six months later than initially scheduled. The postoperative course was complicated by a complete heart block requiring a pacemaker and a prolonged inpatient stay.

Intervention 4

The patient requested a further review when recovered sufficiently from his cardiac surgery a number of months later. He reported feeling well after his surgery with no further episodes of pneumonia. Of note, he reported feeling generally much better on cessation of taking statins. The patient continued to complete his dysphagia rehabilitation programme sporadically and was no longer using the supraglottic swallow as a compensatory technique. A repeat instrumental evaluation of swallowing using FEES was undertaken to guide further management. Main findings from the FEES were as follows:

- Incomplete epiglottic movement;
- Incomplete laryngeal–vestibular closure;
- Penetration across food and fluid consistencies during the swallow;
- Silent aspiration post swallow;
- Supraglottic swallow appeared to enhance swallowing efficiency and safety.

A full and detailed explanation of the swallowing dysfunction was shared with the patient. The management plan after repeat instrumental examination included safe swallowing guidelines, oral hygiene advice and compensatory strategies, with use of the supraglottic swallow in addition to a revised therapeutic plan. The Shaker exercise was now contraindicated due to recent cervical spine injury. The evidence base for the use of expiratory muscle strength training (EMST) to aid cough clearance and submental muscle activity (Wheeler-Hegland et al., 2008) was increasing. More recently, EMST has shown some positive outcomes for HNC patients (Hutcheson, 2017). After confirming his suitability, this intervention was introduced utilizing a standard protocol (see https://emst150.com).

Given our concerns about his ongoing respiratory issues, we referred this man for a specialist review. Just before this, he underwent surgery for an infected upper right molar which had eroded into his maxillary sinus, leaving a 5-mm hole, thus prompting us to suspend his EMST programme but to continue with his other dysphagia therapy exercises.

The respiratory physicians found that, on a lung CT scan, he had a persisting right middle lobe collapse and the presence of extended-spectrum beta-lactamases (ESBLs) (Department of Health, 2014) in his sputum producing *Escherichia coli*, which is resistant to many antibiotics. He was subsequently referred for enhanced airway clearance techniques with the respiratory physiotherapists.

It was explained to the patient that his respiratory issues would probably increase given aspiration-related lung injury and, with increased antibiotics, the more resistant pathogens were likely to emerge. It was also confirmed that, although the tooth infection might be contributing to his upper respiratory tract infections, this was a less likely factor than his known aspiration.

Respiratory investigations and exploration of treatment options continue at the time of writing. It is notable that during these recent respiratory consultations, the patient has reiterated the importance and pleasure that oral intake represents to him and that he does not want to consider enteral feeding.

Patient perspective

> Certainly, my swallowing problems became worse after 4–5 years post-HNC treatment. I am 9 years post-HNC and there is pressure . . . to consider nil by mouth and a feeding tube, but I firmly believe this is a red line for me. Also, even without food and drink in the mouth, there are plenty of bad bacteria in the mouth to aspirate. The NMES treatment I had in the USA did not appear to help noticeably. Perhaps because I was an engineer in my career, I found the FEES very useful in helping me manage my swallowing. I do believe swallowing/ throat exercises do help in improving my swallow.

Follow-up and outcomes

Intervention and regular review for this man are currently ongoing. However, it is unclear how long follow-up should continue. The hope is to reinstate EMST when the patient is medically fit for this intervention, with pre- and post-intervention outcome measures. In the event that there is no change in swallowing function after further intervention, it is likely that the patient will remain under surveillance in partnership with our respiratory colleagues.

This patient's care has been complicated by the number of healthcare services he has accessed within the NHS and independent providers both in the UK and abroad. In addition, regular follow-up was not possible due to his travel commitments and his distance from the treating centre. There is the potential for further deterioration in the future, with a steady decline in swallowing function being reported despite rehabilitative techniques (Hutcheson et al., 2015). A large part of the care of this patient has been in the education of the aetiology and nature of his dysphagia. In line with the National Cancer Survivorship Initiative (NCSI, 2014) patients must be empowered to seek support and play an active role in their rehabilitation.

With regard to changes in swallowing physiology it would appear that this man's swallow has not responded to traditional therapeutic techniques, which is in keeping with the literature (Hutcheson et al., 2015; Langmore et al., 2016). In addition, his response to more novel techniques including NMES is consistent with the findings of the largest clinical trial to date (Langmore et al., 2016). The patient, however, feels that interventions for his swallowing dysfunction are useful and this too is in line with the literature suggesting that patients' QoL may be improved with swallowing interventions (Langmore et al., 2016).

Discussion

Dysphagia is one of the most disabling consequences of the treatment of HNC, resulting in compromised nutrition, aspiration, pneumonia and impaired QoL. The nature and severity of dysphagia for the HNC patient are both complex and have the potential to change over time, depending on the treatments received. With regard to surgery the patient is likely to experience tissue loss with a subsequent impact on range of motion and possible denervation. Short-term side effects include postoperative oedema and pain. Longer-term postoperative complications can result in atrophy and scarring, particularly in combination with radiotherapy. Radiotherapy can also cause both acute and long-term dysphagia and there is now an emerging evidence base for the occurrence of late effects in which new-onset swallowing difficulties occur after several years of functional swallowing (Hutcheson et al., 2012). The late effects of treatment on swallowing can be under-reported and under-recognized (Szczesniak et al., 2014). Swallowing interventions are required at several time points throughout the patient's care and, in line with national and international guidance, SLTs should see HNC patients before their treatment for baseline assessment and counselling, during radiotherapy and for ongoing rehabilitation post-treatment (Department of Health and Ageing South Australia, 2013; NCCN, 2013; Ministry of Health, New Zealand, 2015; British Association of Head and Neck Oncologists, 2016; NICE, 2016). Robust, multi-dimensional, dysphagia outcome measures are essential to provide accurate diagnostic and prognostic information to patients, as well as guiding rehabilitation, and to assess for change over time. For this reason, an increasing number of clinical trials, which address swallowing outcomes, are now following people up over longer periods of time (Owadally et al., 2015; Petkar et al., 2016). Patients should be informed of the potential acute and longer-term risk for dysphagia and therefore be empowered to monitor symptoms, access support and play an active role in their rehabilitation.

References

Bianchi C & Cantarella G. 2011, 'Chronic aspiration without pulmonary complications after partial laryngectomy: long-term follow-up of two cases', *Dysphagia*, 26(3), 332–336.

Bhayani MK, Hutcheson KA, Barringer DA et al. 2013, 'Gastrostomy tube placement in patients with oropharyngeal carcinoma treated with radiotherapy or chemoradiotherapy: factors affecting placement and dependence', *Head & Neck*, 35(11), 1634–1640.

British Association of Head and Neck Oncologists. 2016, *Head and Neck Cancer: Multidisciplinary team guidelines*. London: BAHNO.

Brown TE, Banks MD, Hughes BG, Lin CY, Kenny LM & Bauer JD. 2017, 'Randomised controlled trial of early prophylactic feeding vs. standard care in patients with head and neck cancer', *British Journal of Cancer*, 117(1), 15–24.

Chen AY, Frankowski R, Bishop-Leone J et al. 2001, 'The development and validation of a dysphagia-specific quality-of-life questionnaire for patients with head and neck cancer: the MD Anderson dysphagia inventory', *Archives of Otolaryngology–Head & Neck Surgery*, 127(7), 870–876.

Clavel S, Fortin B, Després P et al. 2011, 'Enteral feeding during chemoradiotherapy for advanced head-and-neck cancer: a single-institution experience using a reactive approach', *International Journal of Radiation Oncology Biology Physics*, 79(3), 763–769.

Department of Health and Ageing, Government of South Australia. 2013, South Australian head and neck cancer pathway; optimising outcomes for all south Australians diagnosed with head and neck cancer, available at: https://www.sahealth.sa.gov.au/wps/wcm/connect/75e97b00417895249786ff67a94f09f9/Head+and+Neck+Cancer+Pathway+FINAL.pdf?MOD=AJPERES&CACHEID=75e97b00417895249786ff67a94f09f9 (accessed 1 July 2017).

Department of Health. (2014) Extended-spectrum beta-lactamases (ESBLs): guidance, data, analysis, available at: https://www.gov.uk/government/collections/extended-spectrum-beta-lactamases-esbls-guidance-data-analysis (accessed 29 December 2017).

Doeltgen SH, Witte U, Gumbley F & Huckabee M. 2009, 'Evaluation of manometric measures during tongue-hold swallows', *American Journal of Speech–Language Pathology*, 18, 65–73.

Fujiu M & Logemann JA. 1996, 'Effect of a tongue-holding maneuver on posterior pharyngeal wall movement during deglutition', *American Journal of Speech-Language Pathology*, 5(1), 23–30.

Hirano M. 1981, '"GRBAS" scale for evaluating the hoarse voice and frequency range of phonation', *Clinical Examination of Voice*, 5, 83–84.

Hirst LJ, Sama A, Carding PN & Wilson JA. 1998, 'Is a 'safe swallow' really safe?', *International Journal of Language and Communication Disorders*, 33(suppl 1), 279–280.

Hutcheson KA. 2017, 'Cough, expiratory training, and chronic aspiration after head and neck radiotherapy', available at: https://clinicaltrials.gov/ct2/show/NCT02662907 (accessed 20 July 2017).

Hutcheson KA, Lewin JS, Barringer DA et al. 2012. 'Late dysphagia after radiotherapy-based treatment of head and neck cancer', *Cancer*, 118(23), 5793–5799.

Hutcheson KA, Yuk MM, Holsinger FC, Gunn GB & Lewin J. 2015, 'Late radiation-associated dysphagia with lower cranial neuropathy in long-term oropharyngeal cancer survivors: video case reports', *Head & Neck*, 37(4), E56–E62.

Hutcheson KA, Barrow MP, Warneke CL et al. 2017a, 'Cough strength and expiratory force in aspirating and nonaspirating postradiation head and neck cancer survivors', *The Laryngoscope*, doi:10.1002/lary.26986 (e-pub ahead of print).

Hutcheson KA, Yuk M, Hubbard R et al. 2017b, Delayed lower cranial neuropathy after oropharyngeal intensity-modulated radiotherapy: A cohort analysis and literature review' *Head & Neck*, 39(8), 1516–1523.

Kraaijenga SAC, van den Brekel, MWM & Hilgers FJM. 2014, 'Current assessment and treatment strategies of dysphagia in head and neck cancer patients: a systematic review of the 2012/13 literature', *Current Opinion in Supportive and Palliative Care*, 8(2), 152.

Lam L & Samman N. 2013, 'Speech and swallowing following tongue cancer surgery and free flap reconstruction–a systematic review', *Oral Oncology*, 49(6), 507–524.

Langmore SE, Terpenning MS, Schork A et al. 1998, 'Predictors of aspiration pneumonia: how important is dysphagia?' *Dysphagia*, 13(2), 69–81.

Langmore SE, McCulloch TM, Krisciunas GP et al. 2016, 'Efficacy of electrical stimulation and exercise for dysphagia in patients with head and neck cancer: a randomized clinical trial', *Head & Neck*, 38, S1.

List MA, Ritter-Sterr C & Lansky SB. 1990, 'A performance status scale for head and neck cancer patients, *Cancer*, 66(3), 564–569.

Logemann JA. 1998, *Manual for the Videofluorographic Study of Swallowing*, 2nd edn, Austin, TX: Pro Ed.

Ministry of Health, New Zealand. 2015, 'National tumour standards', available at: www.health.govt.nz/our-work/diseases-and-conditions/cancer-programme/faster-cancer-treatment-programme/national-tumour-standards (accessed 1 July 2017).

National Cancer Survivorship Initiative. 2013, 'Living with and beyond cancer: taking action to improve outcomes', available at: https://www.gov.uk/government/.../9333-TSO-2900664-NCSI_Report_FINAL.pdf (accessed 29 January 2018).

National Institute for Health and Care Excellence (NICE). 2016, 'Cancer of the upper aerodigestive tract: assessment and management in people aged 16 and over'. Available at: https://www.nice.org.uk/guidance/ng36 (accessed 29 January 2018).

National Comprehensive Cancer Network (NCCN). 2013, 'Guidelines for head and neck cancer', available at: https://www.nccn.org/professionals/ physician_gls/default.aspx#head-and-neck (accessed 29 January 2018).

Owadally W, Hurt C, Timmins H et al. 2015, 'PATHOS: a phase II/III trial of risk-stratified, reduced intensity adjuvant treatment in patients undergoing transoral surgery for Human papillomavirus (HPV) positive oropharyngeal cancer', *BMC Cancer*, 15(1), 602.

Paleri V, Roe JWG, Strojan P et al. 2014, 'Strategies to reduce long-term postchemoradiation dysphagia in patients with head and neck cancer: an evidence-based review', *Head & Neck*, 36(3), 431.

Patterson JM, Hildreth A, McColl E, Carding PN, Hamilton D & Wilson JA. 2011, 'The clinical application of the 100mL water swallow test in head and neck cancer', *Oral Oncology*, 47(3), 180–184.

Patterson JM, McColl E, Carding PN, Hildreth AJ, Kelly C & Wilson JA. 2014, 'Swallowing in the first year after chemoradiotherapy for head and neck cancer: Clinician-and patient-reported outcomes', *Head & Neck*, 36(3), 352–358.

Patterson JM, Brady GC & Roe JW. 2016, Research into the prevention and rehabilitation of dysphagia in head and neck cancer: a UK perspective. *Current Opinion in Otolaryngology & Head and Neck Surgery*, 24(3), 208–214.

Peng KA, Kuan EC, Unger L, Lorentz WC, Wang MB & Lang JC. 2015, 'A swallow preservation protocol improves function for veterans receiving chemoradiation for head and neck cancer', *Otolaryngology, Head and Neck Surgery*, 152(5), 863–867.

Petkar I, Rooney K, Roe JW et al. 2016, 'DARS: a phase III randomised multicentre study of dysphagia-optimised intensity-modulated radiotherapy (Do-IMRT) versus standard intensity-modulated radiotherapy (S-IMRT) in head and neck cancer', *BMC Cancer*, 16(1), 770.

Roe JW, Drinnan MJ, Carding PN, Harrington KJ & Nutting CM. 2014, 'Patient-reported outcomes following parotid-sparing intensity-modulated radiotherapy for head and neck cancer. How important is dysphagia?', *Oral Oncology*, 50(12), 1182–1187.

Shaker R, Kern M, Bardan E et al. 1997, 'Augmentation of deglutitive upper esophageal sphincter opening in the elderly by exercise. *American Journal of Physiology-Gastrointestinal and Liver Physiology*, 272(6), G1518–G1522.

Shaw SM, Flowers H, O'Sullivan B, Hope A, Liu LW & Martino R. 2015, 'The effect of prophylactic percutaneous endoscopic gastrostomy (PEG) tube placement on swallowing and swallow-related outcomes in patients undergoing radiotherapy for head and neck cancer: a systematic review', *Dysphagia*, 30(2), 152–175.

Shune SE, Karnell LH, Karnell MP, Van Daele DJ & Funk GF. 2012, 'Association between severity of dysphagia and survival in patients with head and neck cancer', *Head & Neck*, 34(6), 776–784.

Szczesniak MM, Maclean J, Zhang T, Graham PH & Cook IJ. 2014, 'Persistent dysphagia after head and neck radiotherapy: a common and under-reported complication with significant effect on non-cancer-related mortality', *Clinical Oncology*, 26(11), 697–703.

Virani A, Kunduk M, Fink DS & McWhorter AJ. 2015, 'Effects of two different swallowing exercise regimens during organ-preservation therapies for head and neck cancers on swallowing function', *Head & Neck*, 37(2), 162–170.

Wheeler-Hegland KM, Rosenbek JC & Sapienza CM. 2008, Submental sEMG and hyoid movement during Mendelsohn maneuver, effortful swallow, and expiratory muscle strength training', *Journal of Speech, Language, and Hearing Research*, 51(5), 1072–1087.

7 Dysphagia in an individual with Alzheimer's disease

Margaret Walshe, Éadaoin Flynn and Marion Dolan

Introduction

Dementia is a largely irreversible neurodegenerative condition, characterized by decline in intellectual function. As the condition progresses, individuals with dementia can experience memory loss, language impairment, disorientation, changes in personality, difficulties with activities of daily living, self-neglect, apathy, depression or psychosis, and out-of-character behaviour (Weiner & Lipton 2009).

Types of dementia include vascular dementia (VaD), Lewy body dementia (LBD), frontotemporal dementia (FTD), mixed-type dementia and the most common form, Alzheimer's disease (AD). Dementia is also associated with neurological conditions such as Parkinson's disease.

Individuals with dementia often present with feeding difficulties such as difficulty self-feeding, with problems initiating feeding tasks, transferring food into the mouth and maintaining attention to the feeding task (Chang & Roberts 2011). They may also have dysphagia, most often in the later stages of the illness (Suh, HyangHee & Duk 2009). Alagiakrishnan, Bhanji and Kurian (2013) suggest that dysphagia is present in about 50% of people with dementia across various stages of the disease. The characteristics of dysphagia may vary according to the subtype of dementia. For example, people with LBD and dementia associated with Parkinson's disease are reported to have predominantly pharyngeal phase dysphagia (Londos et al. 2013; Shinagawa et al. 2009), whereas people with AD tend to have oral phase dysfunction (Suh et al. 2009). People with FTD tend to have more changes in taste preferences, eating habits and feeding behaviour than people with AD (Ikeda et al. 2002; Langmore et al. 2007).

The consequences of dysphagia for patients with dementia can include dehydration, malnutrition, weight loss, aspiration pneumonia and death

(Gräsbeck et al. 2003; Hudson, Daubert & Mills 2000; Langmore et al. 2002). There is also a risk of choking with associated mortality.

Individuals with dementia can have other characteristics that influence swallowing such as increased age, reduced physical mobility, poor dentition, dependent feeding and use of medications that can affect swallow function (Smith et al. 2009). The following case report describes the management of dysphagia in a woman with AD-type dementia. This case is not unique but it serves to illustrate the unnecessary use of thickened fluids in the absence of comprehensive objective assessments in people with dementia and dysphagia.

Presenting concerns

HB is a 67-year-old woman with probable AD diagnosed 4 years earlier, when she was aged 63 years. This is early or younger-onset dementia. She is married with three grown-up children who all live away from home. She now resides in a nursing home facility, because her husband found it increasingly difficult to care for her needs at home. On the Clinical Dementia Rating (CDR) Scale (Hughes et al. 1982), in which scores range across 0 (no cognitive decline), 0.5 (questionable dementia), 1 (mild dementia), 2 (moderate dementia) and 3 (severe dementia), H has a CDR score of 2, indicating moderate dementia. She has significant memory loss but shows recognition of her family. She occasionally forgets her daughter's name and confuses her with her own sister. She is typically disorientated in time and is periodically confused regarding place, frequently getting lost when returning to her room at the nursing home. She enjoys watching old movies and listening to classical music. Before the onset of dementia, H was a full-time homemaker and an active member of her local community.

A week before referral to speech and language therapy, H was admitted to the acute hospital with dehydration and an upper respiratory tract infection. Three months previously staff at the nursing home noticed that she had begun to cough intermittently while eating and drinking. They subsequently thickened her fluids to a consistency comparable to a slow moving drink and placed her on a soft moist minced diet, because they were concerned about the risk of choking. H's family were unhappy about this because it meant that outings involving food and drink were now more difficult. Before this, H's eldest daughter took her to the local hairdresser every week and then they both had a light snack at a local café. H and her daughter enjoyed these outings. H occasionally had Sunday lunch with her son and her husband at an old favourite restaurant. Participation in social events remains important for both H and her family.

Clinical findings

On admission to hospital, nursing staff completed the 3-oz water swallow test (De Pippo, Holas & Reding 1992; Suiter & Leder 2008). H did not pass this assessment and the nursing staff administering the test believed that she understood the instruction and was able to self-feed the volume of water from the cup given. Given the low diagnostic accuracy for this screening test in people with dementia (Suiter & Leder 2008), and the fact that diet modification was implemented in the absence of a formal swallowing assessment, the medical team requested the speech and language therapist (SLT) to assess H's swallow function.

A review of the medical notes and discussion with the family, nursing and medical team indicated the following:

- A history of fibromyalgia resulting in widespread pain. As a result of H's cognitive communication impairment, the exact level of pain was difficult to gauge but a low level of pain was suspected at the time of this admission;
- Medication included amitriptyline to treat the pain associated with fibromyalgia, although a Cochrane systematic review (Moore et al. 2015) suggests that this medication may not be effective in treating pain for many people. Typically, the medication is used to treat depression. However, the dosage level used to treat H's pain (15 mg) was possibly insufficient to impact on her mood. She also was prescribed donepezil (Aricept), a cholinesterase inhibitor aimed at preventing the breakdown of acetylcholine with a possible impact on improving cognition and memory;
- H had some reduced mobility in recent months with a tendency to spend a lot of time sitting in her chair or sleeping;
- She had a decreased appetite that may be associated with donepezil and needed encouragement to eat;
- Weight loss—H had lost over 5% of her body weight in the previous three months. This was linked to decreased appetite.

Diagnostic assessment

It was important to determine the nature and extent of H's dysphagia. It was uncertain whether her dehydration was associated with thickened fluids and modified diet, and whether her low mood was related to a change in her ability to participate in social occasions. It was also unclear whether she required thickened fluids for swallowing safety or if other compensatory strategies could be trailed.

H was referred to the multidisciplinary team (MDT) for assessment. She was seen by the gerontologist who trialled an increased dose of amitriptyline for low mood. The dietitian reported that H's total protein, albumin and haemoglobin levels, assessed as biological blood markers, related to malnutrition were within the normal range. The physiotherapist assessed physical function and her risk for falls and aimed to increase physical mobility.

The SLT saw H with her son and daughter in a quiet room off the ward area. H's cognitive communication skills were assessed separately and are not reported here. Her son was concerned that her condition had deteriorated with increased confusion and agitation in recent weeks. It was unclear how much the dehydration and recent infection, as well the change in environment, had contributed to this. Information on the nature of swallowing difficulties observed, changes in appetite, food preferences, eating habits and information on other changes in feeding behaviours were obtained. H was included in the discussion and responded when she could. Her family reported that her loss of appetite and recent weight loss were the most salient points and they believed that this was associated with diet modification. H's daughter and son, with some input from H, provided information on her food preferences. With H's permission, she was observed at mealtime back on the ward.

Mealtime observation

H was observed sitting in her chair at her bedside on the ward eating her dinner. A care attendant sat with her and encouraged H to feed herself. H was calm and not agitated. The curtains were drawn around the bedside to prevent distraction. H's dinner comprised a smooth creamy soup, thickened to the required consistency, mashed potato, pureed carrots and a soft white boneless fish with a sauce. Her dessert was warm rice pudding. Her drink was cranberry juice thickened to the consistency of a slow moving drink. The care assistant identified each food item for H and encouraged her to choose which foods she wished to eat on each occasion. The care assistant encouraged small mouthfuls. H drank the juice reluctantly and complained of feeling thirsty. H became increasingly distracted as the meal progressed, losing interest in the food. She ate approximately half of the meal, which took over 45 minutes to complete. Throughout the meal she had to be discouraged from speaking during eating and swallowing. Mild oral residue was noted in the lateral sulci at the end of the meal.

Clinical swallowing examination

A clinical examination of swallowing was completed later in the afternoon after H had had time to rest. She cooperated fully with the evaluation. She had upper and lower dentures but these were now loose fitting and required a dental review. She had a coated white tongue with a dry oral mucosa. This may have been related to her medications. Amitriptyline is known to cause xerostomia and with the higher dosage (125 mg) this was suspected to increase.

Trials of water at room temperature were used (5 ml × 6) and H was asked to drink a pre-measured volume of 20 ml of water from a cup. At the oral phase there appeared to some difficulty initiating a swallow. This is consistent with AD. H coughed on the pre-measured volume of water and it was suspected that she might have aspirated on this. There was no evidence of overt aspiration on a thicker 'nectar'-type consistency and a set pudding consistency. Solids were not trialled but H had already been observed having dinner that included some minced moist foods without any difficulty. It was decided that biscuits/cookies or dry solid foods might place her at risk of aspiration or choking given her dry oral mucosa and lack of dentition.

Videofluoroscopy

It was decided to complete a videofluoroscopy swallowing study (VFSS) on H, as staff at the nursing home were reluctant to return to normal fluids. Although VFSS can be difficult to complete on people with mid to late stage dementia due to problems sitting still and following instructions, H had no difficulty completing the assessment and engaged well throughout the VFSS exam. She was noted to occasionally talk while eating and placed her hand on the side of her face at one point during the exam (full report and videofluoroscopy extract available online—see Suppl 7.1).

Analysis of the VFSS indicated that H presented with mild oropharyngeal dysphagia (Dysphagia Outcome and Severity Scale Level = 5) (O'Neil et al. 1999), characterized by predominantly oral phase difficulties. The exam indicated that H presented with both motoric and sensory deficits. The most clinically significant symptoms impacting on swallow function included prolonged and disorganized bolus preparation, lingual searching movements and disorganized anterior–posterior lingual movements, with overall difficulty initiating the swallow. These signs were noted across grades of fluids and thicker consistency trials. Airway penetration was recorded on sips of thin liquid and on teaspoons of smooth puree. Penetrated material remained above the vocal folds and was spontaneously ejected from the airway. On one trial of smooth puree material remained above the vocal folds and was not ejected from the airway. Mild residue was noted in the valleculae and pyriform sinus on thin liquids and trials of puree. Retrograde flow through the upper oesophageal sphincter was recorded on one occasion on thin liquids. A possible cricopharyngeal bar was also noted at the level of C5–6, which may have impacted on oesophageal transit.

Therapeutic intervention

Research studies (Foley, Affoo & Martin 2015; Manabe et al. 2017) confirm that certain subtypes of dementia, specifically AD, are associated with increased mortality rates linked to pneumonia. Management of dysphagia and reducing risk of developing aspiration pneumonia are therefore important. Weight loss is also associated with increased mortality (Hanson et al. 2013). Typical compensatory strategies that are used with individuals with dementia include taking small sips or small bite sizes, using a chin-down head posture, using a liquid wash to clear residue following a solid bolus, using a double swallow to clear pharyngeal residue or a finger sweep to clear oral residue. Typically, diets are modified and liquids thickened as a first-line strategy to help improve dysphagia.

Although the immediate effect of thickening fluid in eliminating aspiration is apparent on VFSS in people with dementia, this may not be in the person's best interest in the longer term. Logemann et al. (2008) examined the efficacy of thickened fluids versus chin tuck in a cohort of people with dementia alone, and people with Parkinson's disease with and without dementia. Using VFSS and data on 351 people with dementia alone, participants were less likely to aspirate on 'honey-thick' (3000 cPs) liquids and this was more effective in minimizing aspiration than 'nectar thick' (300 cPs) and chin-tuck posture. However, Robbins et al. (2008) followed up these participants over a three-month period. They found that, although 'honey-thick' liquids eliminated aspiration on VFSS, in the long term people with dementia on the 'honey-thick' fluids had a greater incidence of pneumonia, dehydration, urinary tract infections and fever requiring hospitalization, compared with those on 'nectar-thick' or regular fluids and chin-down posture. This emphasizes the need for long term monitoring of people with dementia on thickened fluids. H does not require thickened fluids here and can revert to normal thin fluids.

Other modifications such as carbonated liquids may have a positive impact, particularly in those with reduced oral and pharyngeal sensation, but they are largely under-investigated in people with dementia (Larsson et al. 2017). We argue here that modification of the consistency of fluid should not be the sole management strategy and, as in H's case, can result in dehydration and a decrease in participation in social activities.

Compensatory strategies and spaced retrieval

Cognitive deficits in dementia mean that implementing compensatory techniques to improve swallowing can be challenging due to difficulty learning new strategies. H should trial some compensatory strategies. Despite the general belief that individuals with dementia are unable to learn anything new, one intervention that shows promise is spaced retrieval (SR), defined by Benigas and Bourgeois (2016, p. 322) as a 'memory training strategy that is used to help people with memory impairment learn, maintain, and recall functional information by targeting implicit memory systems that are relatively unimpaired in persons with dementia'. SR involves the person with dementia verbally rehearsing the response to a priming question (e.g. priming question: 'after you take a drink, what should you do? Response 'I need to swallow twice'). This is practised over increased time intervals.

The SR protocol can be combined with visual aids to enhance learning in people with dementia and dysphagia who have intact reading comprehension skills. Brush and Camp (1998) used a case report to illustrate how SR and a written visual cue were used successfully to teach an older man with dysphagia and moderate dementia (Mini-Mental State Examination [MMSE] score of 19) to take a drink after he had swallowed food. To ensure that any SR intervention continues to be effective with long-term follow-up, it is important that family and care staff are trained in the intervention so that they can continue to monitor progress and maintain the strategies taught to the person with dementia (Hunter, Ward & Camp 2012).

Based on H's dysphagia assessment, MDT findings and an interview with H and her family, recommendations were made on H's transfer back to her local speech and language therapy service (Table 7.1). Environmental modification and support (Brush, Meehan & Calkins 2002; Hellen 2002; Roberts & Durnbaugh 2002) is essential for safe eating and swallowing, as well as improved quality of life. Screening and preventative systems for nutritional care in consultation with the dietitian are also important given that the risk for malnutrition is high in people with AD. Management of H's swallowing requires ongoing input from the MDT as the condition progresses. Training of staff at the nursing home is essential. It is advisable that an SLT and occupational therapist monitor and review H's progress, ideally within an agreed time scales.

Table 7.1 Recommendations for eating, drinking and swallowing for H

1. Small bolus volumes of normal fluids: a Provale® cup should be trialled.
2. Encourage H to feed herself where possible and allow H extra time to feed herself.
3. Sensory enhancement of food and fluids. Trial of carbonated beverages or very cold drinks with the addition of extra flavours.
4. SR trial to teach double swallow and finger sweep of mouth for oral care. If not then frequent oral hygiene and verbal reminders with regard to double swallow.
5. Discourage H from speaking while there is food in her mouth.
6. Facilitate H to select her own food from a menu that contains only suitable foods (avoidance of nuts, foods with hard outer shells, stringy foods, etc.).
7. Small frequent meals to accommodate reduced attention levels, fatigue and distractibility.
8. If H has increased difficulty managing cutlery, then continue to **encourage self-feeding** where possible using finger foods (banana, cubes of soft cheese, small muffins, etc.) as long as these foods are not high-risk foods for H.
9. Focusing on improving the food choices available and content of the midday meal. This is believed to provide the greatest calorie intake.
10. Adapt the mealtime environment with the help of the speech and language therapist and occupational therapist to ensure appropriate cutlery and utensils for a quiet, well-lit, mealtime environment. This environment should provide an opportunity to observe but also interact with individuals.
11. Keep items presented on a plate or tray simple and to a minimum. It is suggested that people with dementia may be overwhelmed by a large number of different items, all presented at once.
12. Presentation of food on a plate is important. Meals should be colourful and easily identified. Food lacking in colour and contrast such as white fish, with white bread, a white sauce and mashed potatoes on a white plate should be avoided.
13. Flexible mealtimes where H can eat when she wants to or when she is less tired and distractible.
14. Checking oral hygiene at the end of a meal.
15. Encourage H to remain in an upright position after eating and drinking to reduce oesophageal reflux.
16. Monitoring of H's fluid intake with regular weighing and nutritional monitoring.
17. Provide opportunities for H to participate in family social occasions that involve eating and drinking for as long as possible.

Follow-up and outcomes

See the timeline of the episode of care (Figure 7.1). H was transferred back to the nursing home and referred on to her local SLT who provided a service to H's nursing home. Challenges included allowing flexibility around mealtimes, because there were constraints linked to changes to routines in the nursing home. Presentation and sensory enhancement of food proved to be adopted easily by staff and enjoyed by H. Self-feeding was also a complete change for staff and, although it did depend on H's physical ability, it did give her more control over food intake.

Discussion

Four basic principles described by Brooker (2004) should direct our management of people with dementia (VIPS): V = the value of human lives regardless of age or cognitive ability; I = an individualised approach acknowledging each person's uniqueness; P = understanding the world from the perspective of the person with dementia; and S = a social environment that supports psychological needs and fosters well-being. Throughout the assessment process these principles were central to evaluating H's dysphagia and designing an intervention programme. It was fortunate that H had strong family support and access to dysphagia and videofluoroscopy services.

The primary take-home messages are that thickening fluids and diet modification should not be the first line of management in people with dysphagia and dementia without careful and thorough assessment, implementing instrumental examination, if possible. The risk of aspiration, malnutrition, dehydration and choking should be minimized while valuing quality of life. The consequences of food and fluid restrictions are significant not only for the person with dementia but also for families. Where possible, the perspective of the person with dementia should be sought. Qualitative research involving people with dementia suggest that they should be involved in mealtime choice and in discussion on feeding where possible (Milte et al. 2017). Early discussions regarding tube feeding are advised. Alternative non-oral tube feeding in people with severe dementia has been greatly debated in recent years in the absence of firm evidence that it prevents aspiration pneumonia or increases quality of life (Royal College of Physicians and British Society of Gastroenterology 2010). Finally, retaining the social environment— continuing to provide opportunities for participation in family social occasions—is vital to retain relationships and promote wellbeing.

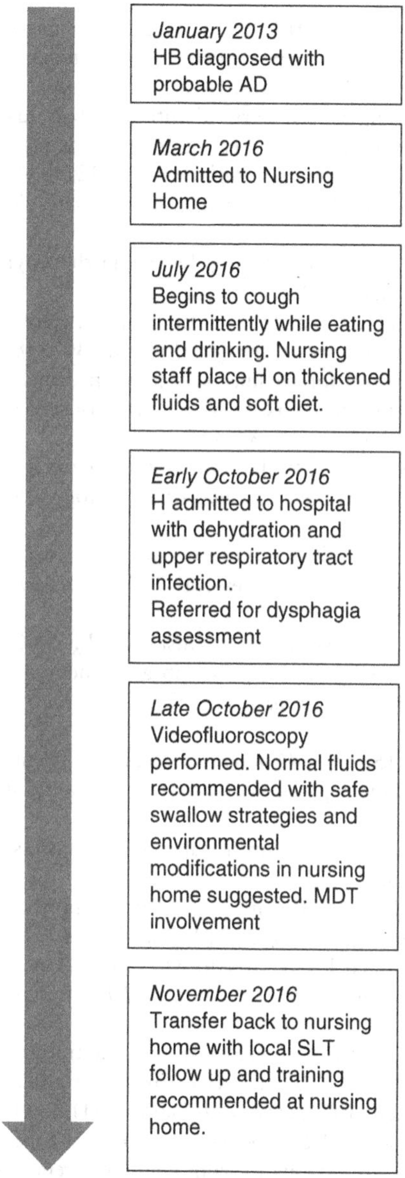

January 2013
HB diagnosed with probable AD

March 2016
Admitted to Nursing Home

July 2016
Begins to cough intermittently while eating and drinking. Nursing staff place H on thickened fluids and soft diet.

Early October 2016
H admitted to hospital with dehydration and upper respiratory tract infection.
Referred for dysphagia assessment

Late October 2016
Videofluoroscopy performed. Normal fluids recommended with safe swallow strategies and environmental modifications in nursing home suggested. MDT involvement

November 2016
Transfer back to nursing home with local SLT follow up and training recommended at nursing home.

Figure 7.1 Timeline of clinical care

References

Alagiakrishnan K, Bhanji RA & Kurian M. 2013, 'Evaluation and management of oropharyngeal dysphagia in different types of dementia: a systematic review', *Archives of Gerontology and Geriatrics*, 56, 1–9.

Benigas JE & Bourgeois M. 2016, 'Using spaced retrieval with external aids to improve use of compensatory strategies during eating for persons with dementia', *American Journal of Speech–Language Pathology*, 25, 321–334.

Brooker D. 2004, 'What is person-centred care in dementia?', *Reviews in Clinical Gerontology*, 13, 215–222.

Brush JA & Camp CJ. 1998, 'Spaced Retrieval during dysphagia therapy: A case study', *Clinical Gerontologist*, 19(2), 96–99.

Brush JA, Meehan RA & Calkins M. 2002, 'Using the environment to improve intake for people with dementia', *Alzheimer's Care Quarterly*, 3. 330–338.

Chang C & Roberts BL. 2011, 'Strategies for feeding patients with dementia: How to individualize assessment and intervention based on observed behavior. *American Journal of Nursing*, 111(4), 36–44.

De Pippo K, Holas MA & Reding MJ. 1992, 'Validation of the 3-oz water swallow test for aspiration following stroke', *Archives of Neurology*, 49, 1259–1261.

Foley N, Affoo R & Martin R. 2015, 'A systematic review and meta analysis examining pneumonia associated mortality in dementia', *Dementia and Geriatric Cognitive Disorders*, 39, 52–67.

Gräsbeck A, Horstmann V, Englund E, Passant U & Gustafsun L. 2003, 'Evaluation of predictors of mortality in frontotemporal dementia—methodological aspects', *International Journal of Geriatric Psychiatry*, 8, 586–593.

Hanson LC, Ersek M, Lin FC & Carey TS. 2013, 'Outcomes of feeding problems in advanced dementia in a nursing home population', *Journal of the American Geriatrics Society*, 61, 1692–1697.

Hellen CR. 2002, 'Doing lunch': A proposal for functional well-being assessment', *Alzheimer's Care Quarterly*, 3, 302–315.

Hudson HM, Daubert CR & Mills RH. 2000, 'The interdependency of protein-energy malnutrition, aging, and dysphagia', *Dysphagia*, 15(1), 31–38.

Hughes CP, Berg L, Danziger WL, Coben LA & Martin RL. 1982, 'A new clinical scale for the staging of dementia', *British Journal of Psychiatry*, 140, 566–572.

Hunter C, Ward L & Camp CJ. 2012, 'Transitioning Spaced retrieval training to care staff in an Australian residential aged care setting for older adults with dementia: a case study approach', *Clinical Gerontologist*, 35(1), 1–14.

Ikeda M, Brown J, Holland AJ, Fukuhara R & Hodges JR. 2002, 'Changes in appetite, food preference, and eating habits in frontotemporal dementia and Alzheimer's disease', *Journal of Neurology, Neurosurgery, and Psychiatry*, 73(4), 371–376.

Langmore SE, Skarupski KA, Park PS & Fries BE. 2002, 'Predictors of aspiration pneumonia in nursing home residents', *Dysphagia*, 17(4), 298–307.

Langmore SE, Olney RK, Lomen-Hoerth C & Miller BL. 2007, 'Dysphagia in patients with frontotemporal lobar dementia', *Archives of Neurology*, 64, 58–62.

Larsson V, Torisson G, Bulow M & Londos E. 2017, 'Effects of carbonated liquid on swallowing dysfunction in dementia with Lewy bodies and Parkinson's disease dementia', *Clinical Interventions in Aging*, 12, 1215–1222.

Logemann JA, Gensler G, Robbins J et al. 2008, 'A randomized study of three interventions for aspiration of thin liquids in patients with dementia or Parkinson's disease' *Journal of Speech, Language and Hearing Research*, 51, 173–183.

Londos E, Hauxsson O, Hirsch I, Janneskog A, Bulow M & Palmqvest S. 2013, 'Dysphagia in Lewy body dementia: A clinical observational study of swallowing function by videofluoroscopy examination', *BMC Neurology*, 13, 140–145.

Manabe T, Mizukami K, Akatsu H et al. 2017, 'Factors associated with pneumonia caused death in older adults with autopsy confirmed dementia', *Internal Medicine*, 56, 907–914.

Milte R, Shulver W, Killington M, Bradley C, Miller M & Crotty M. 2017, 'Struggling to maintain individuality—describing the experience of food in nursing homes for people with dementia', *Archives of Gerontology and Geriatrics*, 72, 52–58.

Moore RA, Derry S, Aldington D, Cole P & Wiffen PJ. 2015, Amitriptyline for fibromyalgia in adults', *Cochrane Database of Systematic Reviews*, 7, CD011824.

O'Neil KH, Purdy M, Falk J & Gallo L. 1999, 'The Dysphagia Outcome and Severity Scale', *Dysphagia*, 14, 139–145.

Roberts S & Durnbaugh T. 2002, 'Enhancing nutrition and eating skills in long term care', *Alzheimer's Care Quarterly*, 3, 316–329.

Robbins J, Gensler G, Hind J et al. 2008, 'Comparison of 2 interventions for liquid aspiration on pneumonia incidence: a randomized trial', *Annals of Internal Medicine*, 148, 509–518. (Erratum in: *Annals of Internal Medicine*, 2008, 148, 715.)

Royal College of Physicians and British Society of Gastroenterology. 2010, *Oral Feeding Difficulties and Dilemmas: A guide to practical care, particularly towards the end of life*. London: Royal College of Physicians.

Shinagawa S, Adachi H, Toyota Y et al. 2009, 'Characteristics of eating and swallowing problems in patients who have dementia with Lewy bodies', *International Psychogeriatrics*, 21, 520–525.

Smith HA, Kindell J, Baldwin RC, Waterman D & Makin AJ. 2009, 'Swallowing problems and dementia in acute hospital settings: practical guidance for the management of dysphagia. *Clinical Medicine*, 9(6), 544–548.

Suh MK, HyangHee K & Duk LM. 2009, 'Dysphagia in patients with dementia: Alzheimer versus vascular', *Alzheimer Disease & Associated Disorders*, 23(2), 178–184.

Suiter D & Leder S. 2008, Clinical utility of the 3-ounce water swallow test. *Dysphagia*, 23, 244–250.

Weiner M & Lipton AF. 2009, *Textbook of Alzheimer's Disease and Other Dementias*, Arlington, VA: American Psychiatric Publishing.

8 Dysphagia associated with respiratory disease

Ulrike Frank and Katrin Frank

Introduction

Chronic obstructive pulmonary disease (COPD) is one of the most common respiratory diseases with an increasing significance for rehabilitation in various clinical settings. The term COPD encompasses a range of different obstructive respiratory diseases such as asthma, chronic bronchitis and emphysema (O'Kane & Groher 2009). Host factors, such as genetic and environmental factors, and, most importantly, exposures to tobacco smoke, occupational dusts and air pollution have been suggested as risk factors for the development of a COPD (Pauwels et al. 2001).

The pathophysiological processes are characterized by chronic inflammation throughout the airways leading to physiological changes, such as mucociliary dysfunction, dilatation and destruction of the respiratory bronchioles, airflow limitation and cardiac dysfunction (McLean 1958; Pauwels et al. 2001). As a consequence, the bronchial pathways collapse during exhalation, leading to obstruction, airway hyperinflation and limitations in alveolar gas exchange. These progressive changes are associated with consistently reduced forced expiratory volumes at 1 second (FEV_1; Table 8.1) and chronic mucus hypersecretion (Pistelli et al. 2003).

Clinically, the disease manifests in frequent but ineffective coughing, high respiratory rates with decreased tidal volume (Rapid Shallow Breathing [RSB]—Yang & Tobin 1991) and progressive phases of exacerbation. The result is a feeling of dyspnoea and exhaustion, and progressive limitations of participation in daily activities as the disease worsens (da Rocha Camargo & de Castro Pereira 2010).

Table 8.1 Spirometric classification of COPD severity based on post-bronchodilator FEV₁

In patients with $FEV_1/FVC <0.70$		
GOLD 1	Mild	$FEV_1 \geq 80\%$ predicted
GOLD 2	Moderate	$50\% \leq FEV_1 <80\%$ predicted
GOLD 3	Severe	$30\% \leq FEV_1 <50\%$ predicted
GOLD 4	Very severe	$FEV_1 <30\%$ predicted or $FEV_1 <50\%$ predicted plus chronic respiratory failure

FEV_1, forced expiratory volume in 1 second; FVC, forced vital capacity.
Global Initiative for Chronic Obstructive Lung Disease (GOLD 2016).

Swallowing dysfunction in patients with COPD

A growing number of research studies have drawn the clinician's attention to difficulties with oral food intake that put COPD patients at risk of malnutrition, pneumonia and reduced quality of life. Generally, patients are more prone to oropharyngeal dysphagia during periods of acute exacerbation (O'Kane & Groher 2009). Concomitant dysphagia can, in turn, increase exacerbations of the disease with rapid deterioration of ventilatory function and hospitalization (Ghannouchi et al. 2016) (Figure 8.1).

Some changes and adaptations within the swallowing sequence due to respiratory impairments are effective compensatory deviations from patterns observed in healthy people, such as an increase in swallowing rates (Nishino et al. 1998; Shaker et al. 1992), longer duration of tongue base contact with the posterior pharyngeal wall (de Deus Chaves et al. 2011) or prolongation of laryngeal vestibule closure when swallowing liquids (Cassiani et al. 2015; Mokhlesi et al. 2002). However, COPD can also result in limited safety of oral food intake due to decreased cough effectiveness and dyscoordinated breathing–swallowing patterns (Gross et al. 2009; Shaker et al. 1992). There is no clear picture, however, about the prevalence of aspiration, with some studies reporting significant aspiration rates (Cvejic et al. 2011; Good-Fraturelli et al. 2000), associated with high respiratory rates, post-swallow penetration and adverse health outcomes (Cvejic et al. 2011), whereas other studies did not find penetration or aspiration events in participants with COPD (Cassiani et al. 2015; de Deus Chaves et al. 2011; Mokhlesi et al. 2002). However, given the limitations in oropharyngeal swallowing function and the inherent pulmonary vulnerability of these patients, instrumental evaluation of aspiration risk is mandatory.

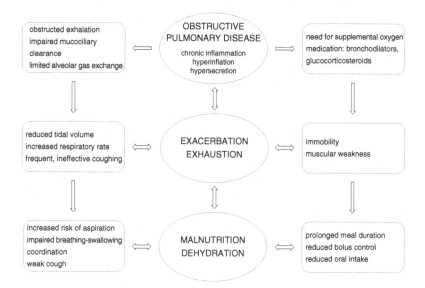

Figure 8.1 Relationships between clinical manifestations of the chronic respiratory disease and swallowing difficulties leading to malnutrition in patients with COPD

The most significant symptoms of dysphagia in COPD patients are ineffective bolus formation and control (Coelho 1987), decreased laryngeal elevation (Mokhlesi et al. 2002) and delayed swallow response time (Good-Fraturelli et al. 2000; Terada et al. 2010). These impairments are probably closely related to orolingual and pharyngeal weakness as a result of age, decreased physical activity and chronic illness (Harris 1997, Lindle et al. 1997). During eating, this leads to significantly prolonged oral and pharyngeal bolus transit times (OTT, PTT) (Coelho 1987), oral residue and bilateral valleculae and pyriform sinus stasis (Good-Fraturelli et al. 2000). Ingestion of solid food is effortful and takes more masticatory cycles, more swallows and increased time compared to age- and gender-matched healthy individuals (Lerbs et al. 2017). Thus, muscle weakness and ineffective mastication of food to smaller particle sizes might be another factor that results in reduced nutrient uptake and malnutrition (Le Révérend et al. 2014).

Decreased tongue strength is associated with prolonged mealtime duration and reduced food and drink intake (Namasivayam et al. 2016). Low saliva swallowing pressure (<26 kPa), in particular, was found to be associated with dysphagia symptoms and nutritional risk in long-term care patients (Namasivayam et al. 2017), with patients using significant proportions (≥88%) of their functional reserve for saliva swallows. Such a decreased range of functional reserve is related to quicker muscle fatigue and greater individual perception of effort (Buchner & deLateur 1991; Burkhead et al. 2007) and has been argued to increase the risk of swallowing impairments in case of decompensation (Nicosia et al. 2000; Robbins et al. 1995).

Recovery from exacerbation and specific muscular resistance training, on the other hand, can increase strength and coordination (Easterling 2013). Coelho (1987) reported that, in his study, participants with COPD often had to rest in the midst of chewing foods due to weakness and dyscoordination of lingual and pharyngeal peristalsis. As strength and endurance recovered, oral transit time (OTT) and PTT approached normal ranges and the promptness of the swallowing reflex improved. This finding highlights consequences that exacerbation-related malnutrition may have on muscle function and the importance of specific interventions to promote recovery.

The following case report illustrates typical challenges and options in the management of swallowing difficulties in patients with chronic obstructive respiratory diseases. It describes the patient's limitations and resources discovered by hypothesis-guided functional assessment and the treatment components for achieving improvements on a functional and participation level.

Presenting concerns and clinical findings

Mr W. was a 68-year-old, retired, post office clerk who was diagnosed with COPD eight years earlier. He stopped smoking 15 years ago, but was a heavy smoker before then. He lived alone in an apartment on the second floor (without a lift/elevator). He had two grown-up children. His daughter, a mother of three children, lived in his neighbourhood. When he was admitted to hospital he was in a state of acute exacerbation with tachypnoea (respiratory rate >29/min) and tachycardia (heart rate >100/min) and he appeared mentally confused. His medication included bronchodilator and glucocorticosteroid treatment, but no long-term oxygen therapy. He had a body mass index (BMI) of 17 (height 180 cm, weight 55 kg). During the previous months, he had had two bronchopulmonary infections and he had lost more than 10% of his body weight. Self-evaluation of his eating difficulties with the Eating Assessment Tool (EAT-10—Belafsky et al. 2008) summed up to a score of 26. Increased effort to eat solid food, to take pills, frequent coughing and stressful perception of eating were rated by him as the most severe problems.

Patient perspective

> My daughter found me in my kitchen and brought me to hospital—I don't really remember how all this happened. I felt very sick and feverish, but I have trouble breathing for so many years now. I have trouble climbing the steps to my apartment, so I go out and buy groceries only once a week, mostly canned soups and ready meals. My mealtimes are quite strenuous for me and they take so long that I give up. I feel that I eat enough but I realize that I have lost a lot of weight and that I get weaker and less active. My daughter helps me with housekeeping when I call her—but I really don't want to be a burden to others. I don't think that my medication is very effective and I am afraid of side effects, besides, I don't remember exactly how and when to use it. I am worried about my weight loss but my biggest problem is my weakness and exhaustion. I would like to enjoy mealtimes more. And I would like to be able to go out and to meet friends.

Diagnostic focus and assessment

Clinical hypotheses and questions

Mr W. was referred to speech and language therapy for evaluation of his capacity and limitations with respect to safe and sufficient oral intake. Based on the clinical presentation and the patient-reported concerns, we hypothesized that the severe respiratory disease with progressive exacerbations led to weakness and dyscoordination of oropharyngeal swallowing, resulting in a state of malnutrition and limited oral intake of nutritious food. Swallowing safety in terms of aspiration risk was unclear and was yet to be clarified. The assessment steps were guided by the following leading questions:

1   Which components of respiratory function and breathing–swallowing coordination that decrease safety and sufficiency of oral intake are impaired? (Cvejic et al. 2011; Gross et al. 2009; Shaker et al. 1992);

2   Is there evidence for impaired oral bolus formation and control, oropharyngeal transport and airway protection during swallowing of different bolus textures? (Coelho 1987; Good-Fraturelli et al. 2000; Namasivayam et al. 2017; Terada et al. 2010);
3   Can compensatory strategies be identified that are effective to reduce exhaustion, avoid aspiration and improve oral intake? (Cassiani et al. 2015; de Deus Chaves et al. 2011; Mokhlesi et al. 2002).

The course of assessments and intervention is illustrated in a timeline in Figure 8.2. Details of the assessment steps are summarized in Figure 8.3.

Functional and behavioural observations during a regular meal situation

The speech and language therapist (SLT) observed Mr W. during a regular lunch meal of potatoes, carrots and bratwurst with meat sauce. Mr W. mashed the potatoes and ate half the meal in 20 minutes. Afterwards, he refused to continue. During eating, the SLT observed an increase of respiratory rate and visible activity of the neck muscles; he began to sweat and his face colour turned increasingly red. Repeatedly, he interrupted eating to rest or to stand up or push back from the table to lean forward with propped up arms ('cart-driver position').

His oral preparatory stage was slow with extensive chewing cycles for each bite of solid food and effortful swallowing. Overt symptoms of food aspiration (coughing, voice change) were not observed. During tooth brushing after the meal, significant residues of food and roughly chewed pieces of sausage spilt into the sink.

Clinical and instrumental respiratory examination

All spirometry measurements (FEV_1, FVC, Tiffeneau index) indicated severe obstructive respiratory dysfunction (GOLD IV—see Table 8.1). Peak cough flow (PCF), a quantitative indicator for cough effectiveness, was 170 l/min and by this only just exceeding the minimum needed to clear secretions from the airway (160 l/min) (Bach & Saporito 1996).

In a sitting position at rest, the patient's thorax was in a hyperinflated inspiratory position, with an elevated position of the shoulders and increased activity of the inspiratory neck muscles, indicating high respiratory effort. His respiratory pattern was characterized by rapid shallow breathing with a respiratory rate >25/min at rest. After repositioning to

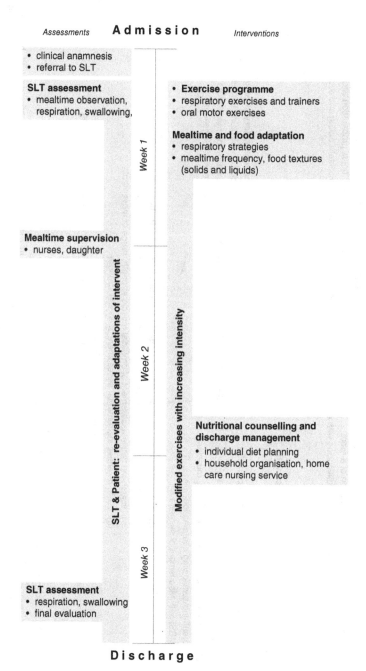

Figure 8.2 Timeline of clinical care

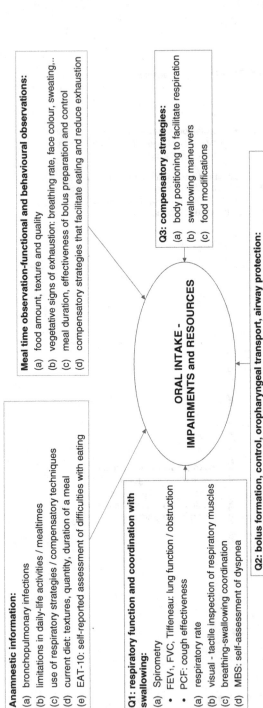

Anamnestic information:

(a) bronchopulmonary infections
(b) limitations in daily-life activities / mealtimes
(c) use of respiratory strategies / compensatory techniques
(d) current diet: textures, quantity, duration of a meal
(e) EAT-10: self-reported assessment of difficulties with eating

Meal time observation-functional and behavioural observations:

(a) food amount, texture and quality
(b) vegetative signs of exhaustion: breathing rate, face colour, sweating,...
(c) meal duration, effectiveness of bolus preparation and control
(d) compensatory strategies that facilitate eating and reduce exhaustion

Q1: respiratory function and coordination with swallowing:

(a) Spirometry
- FEV₁, FVC, Tiffeneau: lung function / obstruction
- PCF: cough effectiveness
(a) respiratory rate
(b) visual - tactile inspection of respiratory muscles
(c) breathing-swallowing coordination
(d) MBS: self-assessment of dyspnea

Q3: compensatory strategies:

(a) body positioning to facilitate respiration
(b) swallowing maneuvers
(c) food modifications

Q2: bolus formation, control, oropharyngeal transport, airway protection:

(a) visual inspection of the oral cavity: dental status, mucosa infections, food residues
(b) visual and tactile assessment of orofacial muscle strength, range of movements
(c) IOPI: objective instrumental assessment of lingual strength
(d) TOMASS: assessment of solid bolus ingestion
(e) VFSS / NZIMES: instrumental assessment of oropharyngeal transport and airway protection

ORAL INTAKE - IMPAIRMENTS and RESOURCES

Figure 8.3 Components of respiratory and swallowing assessment

EAT-10 (Belafsky et al. 2008); Tiffeneau index—FEV₁/FVC, FEV₁, forced expiratory volume in 1 second; FVC, forced vital capacity; IOPI, Iowa Oral Performance Instrument (Robbins et al. 2007); MBS, Modified Borg Scale (Borg 1982); NZIMES, New Zealand Index for Multidisciplinary Evaluation of Swallowing (NZIMES-1) (Hofmayer & Huckabee 2013); PCF, peak cough flow; TOMASS, Test of Masticating and Swallowing Solids (Huckabee et al. 2017); VFSS, videofluoroscopic swallowing study; VC, vital capacity.

the cart-driver position, longer expirations and deeper inspiration were possible.

Breathing–swallowing coordination with saliva swallows and sips of water was assessed by visual inspection of laryngeal swallowing movements and manual palpation of the respiratory cycle on the thorax to determine the phase (inspiration versus expiration) when the swallow occurred. The patient did not deviate from the normal post-swallow expiration pattern (Martin-Harris et al. 2005). Mr W. rated his breathing difficulty as severe (grade 5) at rest and very severe (grade 7) during mealtimes (Modified Borg Scale [MBS]—Borg 1982).

Clinical and instrumental swallowing examination

By visual inspection of the oral cavity, the mucosa appeared dry with gum inflammation and food residue under the tongue and in the cheeks. The tooth status was normal without missing teeth but with poor dental care. Palpatory evaluation revealed a flaccid muscle tone, resulting in weak lip closure, cheek contraction, bite force, tongue protrusion and tongue lateral movements. Assessment of isometric (tongue to palate) and saliva swallow pressures, as measured with the Iowa Oral Performance Instrument (IOPI—Robbins et al. 2007; Youmans & Stierwalt 2006) indicated that the patient used up to 85% of his functional reserve for saliva swallowing (Nicosia et al. 2000; Robbins et al. 1995).

Assessment of solid bolus preparation and swallowing with the Test of Masticating and Swallowing Solids (TOMASS—Huckabee et al. 2017) confirmed limitations in solid bolus ingestion, particularly an increased rate of masticatory cycles and time to finish the cracker.

VFSS assessment of oropharyngeal swallowing function and airway protection was conducted with different consistencies (with (1) liquid: 5 ml and patient-sized cup sip; (2) puree: applesauce; (3) solid: barium bread) and was analysed using the translated German version of the New Zealand Index for Multidisciplinary Evaluation of Swallowing (NZIMES-1—Hofmayer & Huckabee 2013). The patient presented moderate oral dysphagia characterized by poor oral control, resulting in inadequate bolus preparation and post-swallow oral residual. Mild-to-moderate impairments were found in pharyngeal parameters, characterized by inadequate base of tongue (BOT) to posterior pharyngeal wall (PPW) approximation and decreased pharyngeal stripping, resulting in diffuse pharyngeal residue post-swallow. There was no penetration or aspiration of any tested consistencies.

Assessment summary

Several aspects of impaired respiratory and swallowing function were found that limited Mr W.'s oral nutrition. Although we found no evidence for penetration and aspiration at that time, the patient was considered at risk in case of further exacerbation. The most significant impairments were signs of respiratory exhaustion during eating, such as vegetative symptoms, activation of respiratory auxiliary muscles and dyspnoea, which was also confirmed by spirometry measurements. His cough effectiveness was significantly reduced, indicating potential insufficient laryngeal clearance in case of aspiration.

Swallowing function was limited by significant oropharyngeal muscle weakness leading to ineffective bolus preparation, prolonged mealtime duration and—particularly in combination with his respiratory exhaustion—frequent disruptions of eating and low calorie intake.

On the other hand, several resources and helpful compensatory strategies were identified. At the time of examination, no breathing–swallowing dyscoordination and no incidence of aspiration were found. Thus, there was no need for dietary modifications in terms of restriction of food consistencies. Mr W. already used the cart-driver position to facilitate his respiration, however, the frequent application also contributed to mealtime interruptions and an increased exhaustion. Thus, this strategy was not utilized effectively and was considered to be improvable.

Therapeutic focus and assessment

In addition to pharmacological treatment of the underlying COPD, Mr W. received daily physiotherapy and SLT treatment for three weeks in an intensive treatment protocol as one key component of pulmonary rehabilitation and management of his COPD (Skinner 2009). The main aspects of the applied intervention are summarized below. (For an extended list of applied techniques/exercises and their rationale see Tables 8.2 and 8.3.)

The treatment strategy was twofold:

1 *Respiratory therapy*: reduction of respiratory exhaustion by applying methods that regulate respiratory rate and tidal volume, diminish obstruction and facilitate deep exhalation and inhalation. The intended effect was to promote gas exchange and enhance cough effectiveness. Facilitating respiratory strategies were systematically integrated into the mealtime situations with a specific focus on teaching the patient to self-evaluate the utility and effectiveness of the applied methods;

Table 8.2 Respiratory treatment components and intended effects (rationale)

Exercise/technique	Procedures	Rationale
Active cycle of breathing exercises (ACBE) In combination with: • Percussion/ vibration • Positioning	Pursed-lips exhalation • Blowing exhalation with gently closed lips and inflated cheeks ('like the wind blowing') Breathing control • Active and conscious breathing using alternating depth supported by alternating manual contact on the thorax and trunk Deep inhalation—pause—pursed-lips exhalation Sniffing inhalation—pursed-lips exhalation • Two to three short quick inhalations in a row Forced exhalations (huffing) • Inspiration: normal breath; expiration: huffing the air out as if steaming up a mirror	• Creates positive expiratory pressure (PEP) which stabilizes the bronchial system and supports long and sufficient exhalation • Supports thoracic expansion • Inspiratory muscle training • Increased inspiratory volume, increased alveolar gas exchange and cough effectiveness • Supports mucociliary clearance and expectoration of secretions • Facilitates coughing
Respiratory trainers	Secretion management trainers • Handheld training devices that require blowing into a mouthpiece and causing vibrations within the hose that help to mobilize bronchial secretions Respiratory muscle training (RMT): inspiratory muscle training (IMT), expiratory muscle training (EMT) • Inhalation or expiration against a flow-dependent, adjustable, spring-loaded, one-way valve	• Support mobilization of bronchial secretions and expectoration when combined with forced huffing/coughing • RMT: increases activity of the diaphragm and neck and trunk muscles (respiratory auxiliary muscles)—increases tidal volume, cough effectiveness and muscular function
Positioning	Modified cart-driver position • Sitting/standing, bent forward with propped-up arms combined with pursed-lips exhalation	• Repositioning of thorax and shoulder girdle: facilitates deep exhalation and inhalation and reduces exhaustion

Table 8.3 Swallowing treatment components and intended effects (rationale)

Exercise/technique	Procedures	Rationale
Oral motor exercises (OMEs) Against resistance where applicable	• Lip closure • Tongue-to-palate contact • Tongue protrusion and retraction • Jaw opening/closure/masticatory movements • Chin tuck against resistance • Yawn and gargle tasks • Effortful swallows • Masako (tongue-hold) swallows	• Increase strength and range of movement of the orolingual and pharyngeal muscles
Mealtime and food adaptation	• Implementation of respiratory techniques and positioning into the mealtime situation • Cart-driver position combined with pursed-lips exhalation • Increasing frequency and decreasing duration of mealtimes • Five to six smaller mealtimes/day instead of three mealtimes/day • Between-meal snacks Food texture modification/compensatory swallowing techniques • Solids as possible with increasing orolingual and pharyngeal strength—combined with effortful swallowing	• Transfer of techniques and positions that reduce respiratory exhaustion to mealtimes in order to increase time and amount of oral food intake • Smaller and shorter mealtimes reduce exhaustion and increase total food intake • Reduces pressure in single mealtimes • Solid textures, mastication and effortful swallowing supports oropharyngeal muscle function and nutrient uptake
Patient education and discharge management	Together with the dietitian and social worker • Knowledge of appropriate food textures for swallowing • Knowledge about quality and nutrient density of different food types • Recommendations for individual meal planning • Integration of relatives in planning future household organization (e.g. buying groceries, cooking, etc.) • home care nursing service	• Competence in choosing nourishing and high-quality food increases nutritional status • Ensure reliable support for household activities, buying and preparing adequate food • Ensure reliable medical supervision and support

2 *Swallowing therapy*: improved efficiency of oropharyngeal swallowing by conducting a customized oral motor exercise programme to improve strength and coordination of the muscles. Furthermore, the aim was to increase the patient's competence in applying food adaptation strategies and choosing suitable textures of high-quality food, and to establish sustainable family and professional support to ensure adequate nutrition after discharge.

Types and administration of interventions

Active cycle breathing exercises (ACBE)

The respiratory treatment programme (see link to online resources—Table 8.4—included active cycle of breathing exercises [ACBE] and instruction on the use and high-frequent application of respiratory trainers and self-positioning). All exercises, techniques and devices were systematically implemented into the daily structure of the patient to achieve sustainable improvement of his respiratory status after discharge.

ACBE training began with an instruction to the correct performance of the pursed-lips breathing technique, a simple but essential technique for COPD patients *(see Suppl 8.1—Video)*. The positive end-expiratory pressure (PEP) that is established during exhalation by this method stabilizes the bronchial tree, prevents collapse of the bronchial pathway and in this way enables full exhalation and deep inhalation. Mr W. learned this technique quickly and was able to integrate it as a routine exhalation method to all other respiratory exercises and into activities of daily life whenever he felt exhausted. Other ACBE exercises were also learned quickly by the patient and practised during the daily treatment and group therapy sessions.

Respiratory trainers

Mr W. was instructed on the use of training devices for bronchial secretion management (see Suppl 8.2 and 8.3—Videos). He began his training in a $5\times5\times5$ cycle scheme (1 cycle = $5\times$ blows—1 minute break—5 repetitions). One cycle was performed five times a day and was combined with forced huffing or coughing after each cycle to expectorate mobilized secretions (see Suppl 8.4—Video). He was asked to document his contentment with each training session by drawing a sad, neutral or happy smiley face into his calendar. Strong motivation came from self-measurements of oxygenation levels with a

Table 8.4 Results of pre-treatment and post-treatment measurements and normative ranges/cut-off scores

Measurement	Pre-treatment	Post-treatment	Normative values/cut-off scores (95% CI)
Eating Assessment Tool (EAT-10)	26	18	≥3
• Self-reported difficulties with eating			
Spirometry			
FEV₁ (l)	0.65	1.2	2.36
FVC (l)	1.35	2.1	2.81
• Lung function			
PCF (l/min)	170	290	350–550
Tiffeneau index (FEV₁/VC) (%)	29.47	43.3	76.3
Modified Borg Scale (MBS)			
At rest	5 (severe)	3 (moderate)	0 (nothing at all)
• Self-reported breathing difficulty			
During mealtimes	7 (very severe)	3 (moderate)	0 (nothing at all)
Iowa Oral Performance Instrument (IOPI)	85	65	–
Proportion of functional reserve used for saliva swallows (max. isometric pressure tongue to palate—max. saliva swallow pressures) (%)			
Test of Masticating and Swallowing Solids (TOMASS)[a]			
Bites	3	3	2.27 (1.74–2.80)
Masticatory cycles	66	42	36.64 (27.64–45.63)
Swallows	3	2	1.54 (1.10–1.80)
• Effectiveness of solid bolus ingestion			
Total time (s)	75	50	33.55 (27.8–39.29)
Videofluoroscopic swallowing study (VFSS) New Zealand Index for Multidisciplinary Evaluation of Swallowing (NZIMES)	Oral: moderate impairments Pharyngeal: mild–moderate impairments Crico-oesophageal/laryngeal: no impairments		

FEV₁, forced expiratory volume in 1 s; FVC, forced vital capacity; PCF, peak cough flow.

a Age- and gender-matched normative data for TUC Classic™ cracker.

pulse oximeter after each cycle, which helped to structure the exercises and confirmed the improvement to the patient. Respiratory muscle strength training was conducted with specific training devices that require inhalation or expiration against a flow-dependent, adjustable, spring-loaded, one-way valve (see Suppl 8.5 and 8.6—Videos). However, compliance with self-training was low because the patient found the exercises very exhausting. Thus, the protocol was adapted to decreased resistance loads and applied only twice a day.

Positioning

Mr W. already knew and applied the cart-driver position, but his frequent interruptions of eating led to even more exhaustion and reduction of oral intake. Therefore, this position was combined with pursed-lips exhalation to increase its effectiveness (see Suppl 8.8—Video). By this, the patient perceived the facilitating effect more quickly and needed fewer applications of repositioning during the mealtime.

Oral motor exercises

The swallowing treatment programmes (see Table 8.3) included an oral motor exercise (OME) programme comprising movement tasks that enhance strength and coordination of lip closure, tongue-to-palate pressure, tongue protrusion and retraction, masticatory movements of the jaw and pharyngeal motility. When applicable, the tasks included movements against resistance to increase the intensity of the exercises (Robbins et al. 2008). All tasks were instructed by the SLT until the patient could perform them. Afterwards, the patient was given a self-training programme with a selection of five to seven different OMEs that were practised twice a day. As with the respiratory exercises, Mr W. documented his contentment with the training with a sad, neutral or happy smiley. In every therapy session, the SLT checked his ratings and clarified difficulties. Three exercises of the programme were substituted with alternative exercises, and the intensity of the training was increased by systematically adding movements against resistance. Mr W. found the self-evaluation particularly helpful in giving him feedback about his success and rating his own performances increasingly positively.

Mealtime and food adaptation

Food availability was increased by adapting mealtime frequency to five meals a day and offering snacks between meal (Keller et al. 2014). The SLT was present at Mr W.'s midday meals during the first week. Other meals during the first week were supervised by the nursing staff and his daughter. Mr W. learned to apply the modified cart-driver position effectively during mealtimes. Food texture viscosity was extended to more liquids and solids as possible with increasing muscle strength.

Patient education and adaptation of social environment

With a view to future nutrition and household organization, consultation appointments were made with the hospital dietitian and a social worker. During these appointments, strategies for individual diet planning were developed with the patient and his daughter, including education about the quality and nutrient density of different food types that he liked. His daughter also agreed to support Mr W. with buying groceries and preparing food on a regular basis. To ensure medical care and supervision, a daily home care nursing service was organized.

Outcomes

Evaluations of respiratory and swallowing function were repeated (except VFSS) at the end of the three-week therapy period (see Table 8.2). The most significant treatment outcome for Mr W. was his increased spectrum of helpful respiratory and swallowing techniques and food adaptations and that he felt much more competent in applying these methods during mealtimes. In the EAT-10 he still rated 'taking pills' and 'coughing during eating' as severe problems, but all other parameters with respect to solid food intake and stressful eating were rated with reduced severity scores. Likewise, dyspnoea at rest and during eating was rated as only moderate (MBS = 3).

Forced lung volumes and capacities increased during the therapy with an increase of PCF to 290 l/min. This is of particular importance because it indicates his potential for effective airway clearance and protection.

Reorganization from three to five shorter mealtimes a day was perceived as a relief by the patient, and the increased variety of foods and his own competence in choosing the 'right' foods helped him to gain a feeling of autonomy. This significantly improved his enjoyment of food. Positive effects on his improved swallowing and nutritional status were confirmed by a reduction of mealtime duration and oral residue after eating, a significant weight gain, and fewer symptoms of exhaustion during eating and other activities of daily life.

Oral muscular strength and effectiveness of solid bolus ingestion improved, confirmed by reduced buccal pocketing and an increased variety of solid textures that could be integrated into the individual diet plan. Re-evaluation with the IOPI and the TOMASS confirmed this progress, with measurements that approached normal gender- and age-matched ranges of oral performance and use of less functional muscular reserve (65%).

Discussion

The variety and complexity of functional impairments that patients with COPD experience in their activities of daily life require multidisciplinary expertise for adequate management. The treatment of Mr W. integrated respiratory and swallowing treatment, mealtime adaptation and educational approaches. These were implemented into an intensive treatment programme with consideration of training principles that are known to be effective for motor rehabilitation (Maas et al. 2008; Robbins et al. 2008), including training intensity and specificity, but also the early inclusion of self-evaluation strategies to enhance he patient's autonomy and perception of self-effectiveness. The importance of repeated evaluations of treatment suitability for the individual patient is reflected in the fact that some training components had to be reduced because they were rated as too exhausting by the patient. The perception of autonomy and self-effectiveness that could be achieved by the treatment approach combining exercises, compensations, self-evaluation and education should be considered an essential part of pulmonary rehabilitation for sustainable prevention of malnutrition in COPD.

Patient perspective

The treatment during my hospital stay was quite a challenge for me but I appreciate the close interaction with the rehabilitation team. I feel that I could really fix some routines that are helpful to face my limitations and be able to re-act in an effective way. A significant experience for me was that I was asked to evaluate my own progress. That spurred me to stick to my exercises, although there were tough times, especially in the first week when I still felt very sick and weak.

'I never thought that my mealtime routines directly contribute to my respiratory problems but I understand the relationship much better now. I learned a lot about nutritious food and that it is not difficult to prepare tasty meals with little effort. I am aware that my problems will worsen due to the progressive character of my disease. But I feel much better prepared now and I have understood that I have to stick to my medication plan and exercises and seek medical help early to prevent severe worsening and related complications.

Clinical message

The respiratory and swallowing capacities and limitations of COPD patients should be evaluated on a regular basis and treated by an MDT, preferably in an intensive treatment setting, in order to prevent a vicious circle of swallowing dysfunction, malnutrition and exacerbation of the underlying disease.

References

Bach JR & Saporito LR. 1996, 'Criteria for extubation and tracheostomy tube removal for patient with ventilatory failure. A different approach to weaning', *Chest*, 110, 1566–671.

Belafsky PC, Mouadeb DA, Rees CJ et al. 2008, 'Validity and reliability of the Eating Assessment Tool (EAT-10)', *Annals of Otology Rhinology and Laryngology*, 117(12), 919–24.

Borg G. 1982, 'Psychophysical bases of perceived exertion', *Medicine and Science in Sports and Exercise*, 14, 377–81.

Buchner D & deLateur B. 1991, 'The importance of skeletal muscle strength to physical function in older adults,' *Annals of Behavioral Medicine*, 13(3), 91–98.

Burkhead LM, Sapienza CM & Rosenbek JC. 2007, 'Strength-training exercise in dysphagia rehabilitation: principles, procedures, and directions for future research,' *Dysphagia*, 22, 251–65.

Cassiani RA, Santos CM, Baddini-Martinez RO & Dantas RO. 2015, 'Oral and pharyngeal bolus transit in patients with chronic obstructive pulmonary disease', *International Journal of Chronic Obstructive Pulmonary Disease*, 10, 489–96.

Coelho CA. 1987, 'Preliminary findings on the nature of dysphagia in patients with chronic obstructive pulmonary disease', *Dysphagia*, 2, 28–31.

Cvejic L, Harding R, Churchward T et al. 2011, 'Laryngeal penetration and aspiration in individuals with stable COPD', *Respirology*, 16, 269–75.

da Rocha Camargo LAC & de Castro Pereira CA. 2010, 'Dyspnea in COPD: beyond the modified medical research council scale', *Jornal Brasileiro de Pneumologia*, 36(5), 571–8.

de Deus Chaves R, Fernandez de Carvalho CR, Cukier A, Stelmach R & Furquim de Andrade CR. 2011, 'Symptoms of dysphagia in patients with COPD', *Jornal Brasileiro de Pneumologia*, 37(2), 176–83.

Easterling C. 2013, 'Rehabilitative treatment', in: R Shaker, PC Belafsky, GN Postma & C Easterling (eds), *Principles of Deglutition: A multidisciplinary text for swallowing and its disorders*, New York: Springer.

Ghannouchi I, Speyer R, Doma K, Cordier R & Verin E. 2016, 'Swallowing function and chronic respiratory diseases: systematic review', *Respiratory Medicine*, 117, 54–64.

Global Strategy for the Diagnosis, Management and Prevention of COPD. 2016, 'Global Initiative for Chronic Obstructive Lung Disease (GOLD)', available at: http://goldcopd.org/ (accessed 4 August 2017).

Good-Fraturelli MD, Curlee JL & Holle JL. 2000, 'Prevalence and nature of dysphagia in VA patients with COPD referred for videofluoroscopic swallow examination', *Journal of Communication Disorders*, 33(2), 93–110.

Gross RD, Atwood CW, Ross SB, Olszewski JW & Eichhorn KA. 2009, 'The coordination of breathing and swallowing in chronic obstructive pulmonary disease', *American Journal of Respiratory Critical Care Medicine*, 179, 559–65.

Harris T. 1997, 'Muscle mass and strength: relation to function in population studies', *Journal of Nutrition*, 127, 1004S–6S.

Hofmayer A & Huckabee ML. 2013, 'The New Zealand Index for the Multidisciplinary Evaluation of Swallowing (NZIMES)—inter-rater reliability of the translated German version', *DysphagiEforum*, 2, 3–11.

Huckabee ML, McIntosh T, Fuller L et al. 2017, 'The Test of Masticating and Swallowing Solids (TOMASS): reliability, validity and international normative data', *International Journal of Language & Communication Disorders*, DOI 10.1111/1460-6984.12332.

Keller H, Carrier N, Duizer L, Lengyel C, Slaughter S & Steele CM. 2014, 'Making the Most of Mealtimes (M3): grounding mealtime interventions with a conceptual model', *Journal of American Medical Directors Association*, 15(3), 158–61.

Le Révérend BJD, Edelson LR & Loret C. 2014, Anatomical, functional, physiological and behavioural aspects of the development of mastication in early childhood. *British Journal of Nutrition*, 111, 403–414.

Lerbs S, Winkler S & Frank U. 2017, 'Application of the Test of Masticating and Swallowing Solids (TOMASS) in patients with Chronic Obstructive Pulmonary Disease (COPD)', 7th Congress of the European Society for Swallowing Disorders and World Dysphagia Summit, Barcelona, Spain, September.

Lindle RS, Metter FJ, Linch NA, Fleg JL & Fozard JL. 1997, 'Age and gender comparisons of muscle strength in 654 women and men aged 20–93 years', *Journal of Applied Physiology*, 83, 1581–7.

Maas E, Robin DA, Austerman Hula SN et al. 2008, 'Principles of motor learning in treatment of motor speech disorders', *American Journal of Speech Language Pathology*, 17, 277–98.

McLean KH. 1958, 'Bronchiolitis and chronic lung disease', *British Journal of Tuberculosis and Diseases of the Chest*, LII(2), 105–13.

Martin-Harris B, Brodsky MB, Michel Y, Ford CL, Walters B & Heffner J. 2005, 'Breathing and swallowing dynamics across the adult lifespan', *Archives of Otolaryngology, Head and Neck Surgery*, 131, 762–70.

Mokhlesi B, Logemann JA, Rademaker A, Stangl CA & Corbridge T. 2002, 'Oropharyngeal deglutition in stable COPD', *Chest*, 121, 361–9.

Namasivayam AM, Steele CM & Keller H. 2016, 'The effect of tongue strength on meal consumption in long term care', *Clinical Nutrition (Edinburgh)*, 35, 1078–83.

Namasivayam AM, Morrison JM, Steele CM & Keller H. 2017, 'How swallow pressures and dysphagia affect malnutrition and mealtime outcomes in long-term care', *Dysphagia*, DOI 10.1007/s00455-017-9825-z.

Nicosia MA, Hind J, Roecker E et al. 2000, 'Age effects on the temporal evolution of isometric and swallowing pressure', *Journal of Gerontology A*, 55, M634–40.

Nishino T, Hasegawa R, Ide T & Isono S. 1998, 'Hypercapnia enhances the development of coughing during continuous infusion of water into the pharynx', *American Journal of Respiratory Critical Care Medicine*, 157, 815–21.

O'Kane L & Groher M. 2009, 'Oropharyngeal dysphagia in patients with chronic obstructive pulmonary disease: a systematic review', *Revists. CEFAC*, 11(3), 499–506.

Pauwels RA, Buist SA, Calverley PMA, Jenkins CR & Hurd SS, on behalf of the GOLD scientific committee. 2001, 'Global strategy for the diagnosis, management and prevention of chronic obstructive pulmonary disease', *American Journal of Respiratory Critical Care Medicine*, 163, 1256–76.

Pistelli R, Lange P & Miller DL. 2003, 'Determinants of prognosis of COPD in the elderly: mucus hypersecretion, infections, cardiovascular comorbidity', *European Respiratory Journal*, 21(40), 10s–4s.

Robbins J, Levine R, Wood J, Roecker E & Luschei ES. 1995, 'Age effects on lingual pressure generation as a risk factor for dysphagia', *Journal of Gerontology A*, 50, M257–62.

Robbins J, Kays SA, Gangnon RE et al. 2007, 'The effects of lingual exercise in stroke patients with dysphagia', *Archives of Physical and Medical Rehabilitation*, 88, 150–8.

Robbins J, Butler SG, Daniels SK et al. 2008, 'Swallowing and dysphagia rehabilitation: translating principles of neural plasticity into clinically oriented evidence', *Journal of Speech, Language, and Hearing Research*, 51, 276–300.

Shaker R, Li Q, Ren J, Townsend WF, Dodds WJ & Martin BJ. 1992, 'Coordination of deglutition and phases of respiration: effect of aging, tachypnea, bolus volume, and chronic obstructive pulmonary disease', *American Journal of Physiology*, 263, G750–5.

Skinner M. 2009, 'Strength and endurance exercise endorsed for people with COPD', *Physical Therapy Reviews*, 14(6), 418–19.

Terada K, Muro S, Ohara T et al. 2010, 'Abnormal swallowing reflex and COPD exacerbations', *Chest*, 137(2), 326–32.

Yang KL & Tobin MJ. 1991, 'A prospective study in indexes predicting the outcome of trials of weaning from mechanical ventilation', *New England Journal of Medicine*, 324(21), 1445–50.

Youmans SR & Stierwalt JAG. 2006, 'Measures of tongue function related to normal swallowing', *Dysphagia*, 21, 102–11.

9 Multidisciplinary management of paediatric dysphagia

Paige Thomas, Sasha Adams and Maggie-Lee Huckabee

Introduction

Management of dysphagia in paediatrics is complex, demanding not only scrutiny of anatomy and pathophysiology, but also a very careful evaluation of contextual factors that influence presentation of dysphagia and progression towards oral intake. The need for collaborative multidisciplinary management is clear, evidenced by the prominence of reports describing structured feeding clinic areas in the literature. This chapter discusses the unique paediatric case of Holly and her grandmother, Suzy. Crucial messages are portrayed regarding the need for family support and collaboration between professionals in clinical practice.

Oculo-auriculovertebral spectrum (OAVS), often referred to as Goldenhar's syndrome, is a congenital disorder characterized by the potential for dysmorphologies of oral–facial structures, as well as defects of the heart, kidneys and central nervous system, derived from developmental disruption to the first and second brachial arches (Bogusiak et al., 2017). Prevalence of the disorder is poorly defined, with estimations ranging from 1:3500 births to 1:25,000 births (Digilio et al., 2008). As with most congenital conditions, presentation can range from barely noticeable facial asymmetry to very pronounced facial defects, with more or less severe abnormalities of internal organs and/or the skeleton. Yokochi et al. (1997) commented that, although feeding problems related to facial defects are common, long-term tube feeding is not reported to be characteristic of the disorder. This group consequently provided a small case series report of tube feeding in OAVS.

More critical to the presentation of this case than the actual diagnosis is the manner in which the multidisciplinary team engaged both with each other and with the family. Collaboration between members of a multidisciplinary team is critical when providing care for complex paediatric cases (Miller et al., 2001). Importantly, caregivers of children with chronic illness should be integral members of this multidisciplinary team. This allows caregivers to feel as though they are partners in caring for their child, limit their feelings of loss of control and uncertainty, and ensure that they have all the information pertaining to their child's care (Fisher, 2001). Parents of children in paediatric health-care settings respond well to a collaborative relationship, which is centred on trust and communication between parent and clinician (MacKean, Thurston & Scott, 2005). Inclusion of caregivers in the provision of paediatric care may also help to reduce the adverse effects of a harmful parent–child relationship. Munchausen-by-proxy is a syndrome in which a caregiver elicits or exaggerates the symptoms of a child's illness to achieve some secondary gain. There is a spectrum of severity of Munchausen-by-proxy which in the most severe cases involves a caregiver physically harming their child in a manner that is not recognized as abuse to receive medical attention. Although in mild cases the child is not physically harmed by their caregiver, creating a reliance on the caregiver and medical system can affect a child's emotional and physical development (Roth, 1990).

The case that follows details the management of a young girl with OAVS whose long-term tube feeding was inconsistent with functional physiology. This case highlights the need for multidisciplinary inclusion and management, not primarily of the child's swallowing, but also of the relationship between the mother and the child.

Presenting concerns

Holly was 9 years old when she was referred by her physician to a specialist dysphagia rehabilitation clinic. She was diagnosed with probable OAVS as an infant. The presentation of structural deficits was considered very mild in Holly, with minimal asymmetry of low-set ears as the only structural abnormality of the head and neck, and pulmonary artery stenosis as the only abnormality of internal organs.

Despite the mild presentation of structural abnormalities, at birth she presented functional swallowing issues and chronic aspiration, resulting in eventual placement of a percutaneous endoscopic gastrostomy (PEG) for all nutrition and hydration. At age three, she underwent cardiac surgery to widen pulmonary arteries, which resulted in damage to the recurrent laryngeal nerve and consequent unilateral vocal fold paralysis (Hamdan et al., 2002). This left her with a breathy and rough vocal quality. Holly also had some minor developmental and learning delays. She developed mild cylindrical bronchiectasis, which affects the movement of lungs and ability to clear secretions (Pasteur et al., 2000), resulting in a chronic cough and intermittent pneumonia. Cranial nerve examinations in the early years of Holly's life revealed compromise of cranial nerves IX, X and XII.

Reports from the referring health-care team and discussion with Suzy revealed a discord between perception of the severity and the actuality of Holly's illness. Suzy expressed frequent concern that her granddaughter's illness was more severe than recognized by health professionals and that she was not respected as a member of the health-care team despite being the person who spent the most time with Holly. Referring information from the health-care team presented Suzy as a highly invested caregiver, but one who was obstructive to resolving medical issues. There were concerns about the level of inter-dependence between Holly and her grandmother. This included Suzy not allowing Holly to bathe herself and Holly waking up crying in the night to be fed, both atypical developmental behaviours for a child aged nine years. Of greater concern were reports from various medical professionals suggesting that Holly underwent medical procedures at Suzy's insistence which would otherwise have been managed more conservatively. Suzy was also reported to change medical providers if she did not agree with their professional opinion and was not compliant with suggestions from health professionals. For example, following assessment at age eight, the multidisciplinary team strongly recommended implementation of a protocol similar to the Frazier free water protocol (Panther, 2005) to improve the quality of life and begin transition to an oral diet. Reportedly, Suzy ceased the free water protocol on several occasions without seeking further professional advice when Holly developed any cough, because she attributed this to aspiration pneumonia. Pneumonia was not confirmed, and coughing was considered to be due to long-standing bronchiectasis (Pasteur et al., 2000). From a report from the medical team, management of this child had proven ethically challenging, with concerns of significant secondary gain obtained by the grandmother with prolongation of Holly's disability.

Clinical focus and assessment

To ensure that Holly was an appropriate referral to the specialist rehabilitation clinic, several steps were undertaken. Holly underwent a videofluoroscopic swallowing study (VFSS) by a local speech and language therapist (SLT) to provide current information with regard to her swallowing ability (see Suppl Video 9.1). The study included only liquid and thin puree textures. On a report, the therapist also attempted to evaluate oral trials with both water and puree. Initially, intake appeared to be tolerated without difficulty, by further trials were ceased at Suzy's request.

The VFSS was interpreted by the treating clinicians at the specialist clinic. Given that Holly had been PEG fed since birth with only a few attempts at oral intake, the results were surprising. The VFSS revealed quite mild dysphagia, characterized by slightly reduced pharyngeal motility with diffuse post-swallow residual. There were no overt signs of aspiration on any consistency, but one instance of trace penetration on thin liquid, which cleared during the swallow. As penetration during swallowing is seen in approximately 11.4% of healthy individuals (Allen et al., 2010), this was not considered remarkable in a child who has been tube fed for the past nine years. Throughout the study, Holly burped frequently, which the therapists hypothesized was due to swallowing dyscoordination resulting in an increased intake of air.

It was clear from this assessment that Holly's swallowing function had improved dramatically since birth, and rehabilitation to a full oral diet was both appropriate and physiologically achievable. Consequently, after a discussion, it was recommended by the medical team, together with clinicians at the specialty clinic, that Holly receive intensive therapy to transition her to oral nutrition and hydration.

In anticipation of Holly's intensive treatment programme, considerable discussion occurred among the specialist centre personnel, the local multidisciplinary team and Holly's grandmother. It was important that all parties, particularly Holly and her grandmother, agreed to a goal of oral intake and eventual removal of Holly's PEG. Effective and consistent communication between team members was vital to providing an informed assessment of Holly's function and overcoming barriers to success (Leonard et al., 2004). Concerns were raised regarding Suzy's resistance to oral feeding for Holly. Suzy expressed being excited about the opportunity to attend a 'specialist clinic' and ultimately removing Holly's PEG, but she agreed that she would need support to address her anxiety around Holly eating. Consequently, an integral component of the intensive treatment programme would include counselling with a psychologist to address these critical issues and aid transition from PEG to oral feeding.

Diagnostic focus and assessment

As the instrumental diagnostic assessment was completed before the treatment programme, the initial assessment of the intensive programme focused on a review of the VFSS findings with Holly and Suzy, a direct cranial nerve examination, evaluation of oral trials, and discussion about Holly and Suzy's perceptions of swallowing ability and their motivation for eventual PEG tube removal. The previous instrumental assessment revealed only mild dysphagia and no evidence of aspiration on any texture. These findings were consistent with presentation on clinical examination in the clinic. The cranial nerve examination demonstrated improvements from previously reported examinations, with no apparent abnormalities to cranial nerves V, VII, IX, X and XII, with the single exception of Holly's hoarse vocal quality. Holly consumed three small sips of water without apparent difficulty—single, prompt swallows after intake with no wet dysphonia or coughing. Further oral trials were terminated because Suzy expressed anxiety.

Holly's grandmother reported that Holly had suffered from multiple chest infections recently; as a result, she was afraid to push oral intake. She additionally reported that Holly often has a cough that occurs throughout the day and becomes worse a night, indicating that the persistent coughing was not likely to be due to an aspiration event. Furthermore, medical records reported no chest infections in the past two years. These issues were discussed in the first session and the agreed goal of moving towards oral intake was again addressed. It was emphasized that, in order for Holly to be successful, Suzy would need to commit to this goal and work with the team to manage her anxiety.

Therapeutic focus and assessment

The structure and focus of the intensive therapy were developed with Holly, Suzy, a consulting psychologist and the clinicians at the clinic. Holly and Suzy were scheduled to attend twice-daily sessions for swallowing rehabilitation as well as daily psychology sessions, five days per week for two weeks. This intensive programme was considered necessary to ensure uninterrupted transition to oral intake in the perceived 'safe' context of the specialty clinic, with support provided to Holly's caregiver to manage her anxiety and address personal issues that may be impacting her reluctance to allow Holly to move forward.

Swallowing management consisted of using surface electromyography (sEMG) biofeedback to encourage swallowing 'skill' (Huckabee & Macrae, 2014). In many respects, the task was a placebo, providing a focused treatment, first with dry swallows, through which both Holly and Suzy gained more confidence in Holly's swallowing ability before transitioning to bolus swallows. During training sessions, collective activity of the submental muscles was displayed as a time by amplitude waveform on a computer monitor. A 'target box' was randomly placed in each 30-second screen sweep. To achieve success, Holly had to adapt the strength and timing of each swallow such that the peak of muscle activity fell within the target box. This therapy was presented to Holly as a video game—the target was a picture of Holly's face and the leading edge of the waveform was represented by a variety of different foods, from which Holly could choose. Thus, the therapeutic task involved Holly swallowing with sufficient motor control that she put the food into her mouth in the game. This task salience helped to keep Holly interested in therapy.

The skill training blocks were interspersed with ingesting food of varying consistencies. Holly dictated the type of food eaten; consistencies were varied to allow Holly to experience texture differences during mastication. Foods ranged from liquid and puree foods in week 1 to solid and mixed consistencies in week 2. Increasing texture alters the timing, number of cycles and duration of mastication (Steele et al., 2015), and provided greater sensory feedback to a system that had been deprived of oral intake. In healthy individuals, some of a mixed consistency bolus may reach the level of the hypopharynx before swallowing onset (Saitoh et al., 2007). This suggests that mixed consistencies are more challenging to consume.

Whenever appropriate, the therapists and Suzy would share food with Holly to begin to normalize the process of eating and sharing food. Suzy reported that, to protect Holly, food was a taboo subject in their home, with family members forbidden to prepare or eat food around Holly. Holly's two older siblings were required to eat dinner in their respective bedrooms. Thus, normalizing the mealtime environment was considered crucial. Including Suzy in the therapy also allowed her to feel a sense of control of the outcomes and allowed her to experience the progress that Holly was making, so that she could continue to facilitate these changes once they returned home. This feeling of control was critical for Suzy, due to her very close relationship with Holly and their somewhat distorted relationship with oral intake. Therapy included lessons on using utensils and monitoring food temperatures, because these were new experiences for Holly. Holly also expressed interest in meal preparation, which therapists encouraged on the return home to continue to remove the taboo that had been placed on food.

Psychologists were an integral part of the multidisciplinary team for this case. Daily sessions with psychologists were designed to help Holly gain independence from Suzy. This was a significant factor in altering the pair's excessively dependent relationship. Part of the psychological therapy included encouraging Holly to have the opportunity to perform tasks that children of her age should be doing independently, such as bathing herself, selecting foods she wanted to eat and appropriately asserting her independence. Suzy was encouraged to explore her anxiety surrounding Holly's care and what it would signify to her if Holly returned to a normal diet, and was no longer 'disabled'. What would she gain? And what would she lose?

There was a minor setback at the beginning of week 2 of therapy when Suzy believed that Holly was beginning to 'sound rattily' and develop a chest infection. The SLTs noted no evidence of a change in Holly's breathing, unusual coughing or an increase in temperature, and from this determined that a chest infection was unlikely. This provided a valuable teaching moment for Suzy and again demonstrated the importance of family involvement in a child's care. Suzy was able to observe that these symptoms did not develop into anything more serious and was provided with more information about the warning signs of aspiration pneumonia.

In week 2 of therapy, in consultation with Holly's dietitian, discontinuation of PEG feedings was recommended. The rationale was to allow Holly to experience hunger and eat orally for nutrition while still having the safety option of PEG feeding if necessary. Although generally compliant with withholding PEG feedings during the day, Suzy continued to provide Holly with routine PEG feeds at night. She reported that Holly was tired and did not want to eat dinner or that it was difficult to provide a suitable meal for Holly. Suzy also reported that she was concerned that Holly would lose weight; this was addressed with the dietitian who had confidence that any weight loss over this period would not be sufficiently substantial to have a detrimental effect. The psychologists working with Holly and Suzy reported that this inability to comply with the therapy protocol was probably due to the reliance between Holly and her grandmother, and the special bonding time that night-time feeds provided. Multidisciplinary perspectives allowed for increased rationale for continuation of therapy and provided insight into the motivation behind discontinuation. This strong collaboration allowed clinicians to push the intended therapy protocol without fear that it may be detrimental to Holly's health.

Progress

Swallowing precision was measured through sEMG, with a measure of the distance from the target box recorded for all swallows. Throughout the training, Holly's control of her swallowing increased, as evidenced by a smaller distance from the target and larger number of successful attempts at hitting the target in later sessions. Initially during treatment, Holly was taking in excess air while eating, evidenced by an unusually high amount of eructation during sessions. This reduced over time as Holly became more aware of the size of her bolus and swallowing movements necessary for efficient swallowing.

More importantly, the types of foods that Holly felt comfortable eating changed rapidly; this included crunchy foods and mixed consistencies by the end of the first week. Suzy reported that at the end of week 1 she was pleased with Holly's progress and that she had begun informing close family members that Holly was able to eat. Suzy did express that she did not want to tell too many people about Holly's ability to eat different foods because she was concerned that people would suspect that she was feigning Holly's disability in order to profit. Her identification and verbalisation of this possibility were considered significant steps towards recognition of her role in Holly's persisting disability. Clinicians encouraged her to share Holly's success, in part to provide some safeguard against returning to non-oral status after the intensive treatment programme. One of the foods that Holly had reported wanting to eat was pizza; this was achieved in her final session with a 'pizza party', with the clinicians, grandmother and Holly all sharing pizza. Holly appeared to enjoy being able to share this experience with the people who she had become close with, just as many children would at parties or special events.

Follow-up and outcomes

As there were concerns that Suzy would not remain compliant after returning home, therapists called the family daily for two weeks, then weekly for the remainder of the month. In these phone calls, the therapists would enquire about the types of foods that Holly was eating, the settings in which she was consuming these foods, and the frequency of her receiving PEG feeding. The therapists would also provide encouragement that Holly was successfully managing the different varieties of food and that Suzy was effectively encouraging Holly to attempt various foods in different settings.

It was suggested by the extended health-care team that the family continue to allow Holly to consume adequate nutrition without the use of the PEG for one month before it was removed. Suzy continued to express concern about Holly being too tired to eat at night. High-density nutrient supplement drinks gave them an easy alternative to PEG feeding. One week after their return home, Suzy contacted the school to tell them that Holly could eat the foods that she had packed for her lunch but nothing else. These would include soft consistency foods, because Suzy was still concerned that Holly needed special consistencies of food. However, allowing Holly to eat while at school, and allowing her success to be witnessed by others, was a major achievement for Suzy.

During the second week after Holly's return home she spent a day in hospital. This was due to Suzy's report that she was 'chesty' and could not stop coughing. The doctors reassured her that Holly's airway was completely clear and the cough was more likely due to an upper airway issue such as a common cold than to aspiration pneumonia. While in hospital, the dietitian reiterated the importance of weaning Holly from the PEG feeds. After one month, the multidisciplinary team recommended removal of Holly's PEG tube. This occurred without any complications or resistance from Suzy.

One year post-therapy, therapists contacted the family to assess Holly's progress. Suzy reported that, after removal of the PEG, Holly had experienced many firsts such as eating birthday cake at her birthday party, being allowed full access to any food that she wanted in the fridge and participating in cooking meals that they could eat together. Suzy looked at these times with excitement and appeared to be genuinely joyful about her granddaughter being able to participate in normal activities.

Discussion

Management of paediatric dysphagia often involves an equally shared focus on the child and the caretaker. Most often, focus on the family is appropriately limited to education, encouragement, easing anxiety and celebrating successes. Anxiety surrounding initiation of oral feeding may sometimes go well beyond a normal response to a difficult situation and stifle the potential for recovery. It is vital to work with patients and their families in order to create a treatment plan that is achievable for them. The free water protocol was recommended for Holly but Suzy's anxiety meant that this was not an achievable task.

If Suzy had had a clear idea of what an adverse reaction would look like and how this would differ from her baseline pulmonary function through ongoing support and education, she may have been more likely to tolerate this step forward, knowing that it was not detrimental. The ultimate success of Holly's treatment was probably due in part to the intensity of treatment, offering the possibility of dealing with and modifying behaviours of both the child and the caregiver promptly and efficiently.

Even less frequently, the psychological needs of the caretaker may overshadow those of the child, with subtle secondary gains providing a road block to progress. This was a major consideration in this case. Two observations in particular raised concerns. Holly became very anxious around Suzy when trialling foods with the therapist. However, this was not observed when Suzy was not in the session, and reports by others suggested that Holly did not appear to have anxiety around trying foods alone. Suzy appeared to receive secondary gain from her granddaughter's condition through significant online donations, frequent media coverage and additional social support from her community. Suzy had a very strong relationship with Holly, and appeared to favour her over Holly's two siblings who were also in her care. This was apparent from the dismissive comments and lack of regard for the other children when they came into treatment sessions. These traits align with those of caregivers with mild Munchausen-by-proxy syndrome (Roth, 1990). Although Suzy received financial and possible psychological gain from her granddaughter's illness, she did not appear to intentionally harm Holly as is often the case with Munchausen-by-proxy. Indeed, she appeared superficially to be committed to Holly's wellbeing. However, her failure to follow medical advice and continued insistence on non-oral feeding in a child with resolved developmental swallowing impairment raises ethical concerns. It was very clear that psychological support for both Holly and Suzy was the more critical component to the management of Holly's dysphagia.

Close collaboration with members of the multidisciplinary team is paramount. When working with Holly's local SLT, paediatrician, dietitian and psychologists closely, appropriate steps for Holly's care could be determined with a strong rationale. With all of the professionals working towards the common goal of PEG tube removal, Suzy was not able to take one professional's advice from one context and use that to oppose another professional. More importantly, all were able to acknowledge her anxiety and then promptly refocus her back to this goal.

This meant that the therapy continued to run smoothly as Suzy was confident in the advice.

This case is unique in that it represents a situation in which the psychological needs of the caretaker overshadowed the physiological impairment of the child. However, it highlights well the importance of extending the therapeutic focus well beyond the patient. The lessons learned based on the case of Holly and Suzy can be adapted to many cases, helping clinicians to provide the best possible care and fulfil the client's potential.

References

Allen JE, White CJ, Leonard RJ & Belafsky PC. 2010, 'Prevalence of penetration and aspiration on videofluoroscopy in normal individuals without dysphagia', *Otolaryngology—Head and Neck Surgery*, 142(2), 208–213.

Bogusiak K, Puch A & Arkuszewski P. 2017, 'Goldenhar syndrome: current perspectives. *World Journal of Pediatrics*, 13(5), 405–415.

Digilio MC, Calzolari F, Capolino R et al. 2008, 'Congenital heart defects in patients with oculo-auriculo-vertebral spectrum (Goldenhar syndrome)', *American Journal Medical Genetics*, 146A(14), 1815–1819.

Fisher HR. 2001, 'The needs of parents with chronically sick children: a literature review', *Journal of Advanced Nursing*, 36(4), 600–607.

Hamdan AL, Moukarbel RV, Farhat F & Obeid M. 2002, 'Vocal cord paralysis after open-heart surgery', *European Journal of Cardio-thoracic Surgery*, 21(4), 671–674.

Huckabee ML & Macrae P. 2014, 'Rethinking rehab: skill based training for swallowing impairment', *SIG 13 Perspectives on Swallowing and Swallowing Disorders (Dysphagia)*, 23, 46–53.

Leonard M, Graham S & Bonacum D. 2004, 'The human factor: the critical importance of effective teamwork and communication in providing safe care', *Quality and Safety in Health Care*, 13(suppl 1), i85–90.

MacKean GL, Thurston WE & Scott CM. 2005, Bridging the divide between families and health professionals' perspectives on family-centred care. *Health Expectations*, 8(1), 74–85.

Miller CK, Burklow KA, Santoro K, Kirby E, Mason D & Rudolph CD. 2001, 'An interdisciplinary team approach to the management of pediatric feeding and swallowing disorders', *Children's Health Care*, 30(3), 201–218.

Panther K. 2005, 'The Frazier free water protocol', *Perspectives on Swallowing and Swallowing Disorders (Dysphagia)*, 14(1), 4–9.

Pasteur MC, Helliwell SM, Houghton SJ et al. 2000, 'An investigation into causative factors in patients with bronchiectasis', *American Journal of Respiratory and Critical Care Medicine*, 162(4,) 1277–1284.

Roth D. 1990. 'How "mild" is mild Munchausen syndrome by proxy?', *Israel Journal of Psychiatry and Related Sciences*, 27(3), 160–167.

Saitoh E, Shibata S, Matsuo K, Baba M, Fujii W & Palmer JB. 2007, Chewing and food consistency: effects on bolus transport and swallow initiation. *Dysphagia*, 22(2), 100–107.

Steele CM, Alsanei WA, Ayanikalath S et al. 2015, 'The influence of food texture and liquid consistency modification on swallowing physiology and function: a systematic review', *Dysphagia*, 30(1), 2–16.

Yokochi K, Terasawa SI, Kono C & Fujishima I. 1997, 'Dysphagia in children with oculo-auriculo-vertebral spectrum', *Dysphagia*, 12(4), 222–225.

10 Beyond case reports

Putting the single-subject design to work

Joseph Murray

Introduction

In this compilation of clinical cases the reader has had the opportunity to inspect interactions between clinicians and patients that are likely familiar and may represent the daily struggle many of us experience as we attempt to deliver an intervention that will yield a meaningful outcome. Paired with the struggle are external pressures to deliver care with an "evidence base" that can generate a fear in practicing clinicians that the evidence available may be inapplicable or inappropriate for their individual patient (Sackett, 1997). Many feel that practicing "within the evidence" is inexact and difficult to replicate in a clinical setting and that the only valuable evidence comes in the form of large-scale, randomly controlled trials, systematic reviews and meta-analysis (Rogers & Graham, 2008). These same practitioners may be surprised to find that the daily effort of interacting with single patients, if carefully planned and executed, allows for scientific inspection equal to the most powerful forms of evidence in the world of medical research (Guyatte et al., 1988).

Recently there has been an increase in emphasis on designing and delivering "patient-centered care" and with it comes a connected movement to engage and master small, single-subject research studies. Taming the lexicon that is often used when describing these efforts is the first step closer to understanding the process and producing your own work. The terms "case report," "case study," "single-subject study" and "*n*-of-1 study" are frequently but incorrectly used synonymously because they are distinctly different in their intention and execution (Krasny-Pacini & Evans, 2018). Readers must first familiarize themselves with the terminology related to studying a single subject.

Case report

As discussed in Chapter 1, a case report is typically sourced from clinical practice and describes and analyzes the diagnosis, treatment course and response of a patient. Case reports typically articulate a unique clinical presentation that may inform the field of an unknown condition or set of symptoms. The report may also describe an unexpected response to treatment or progression of symptoms after treatment, which indicates a novel therapeutic effect or, alternately, an unexpected adverse effect of treatment.

Case reports can also describe how diagnosis or treatment for known diseases can be enhanced by innovative technologies. They may also describe hazards or potential adverse outcomes associated with new treatments.

A case report is not expected to influence a field's approach to assessing and treating patients in the way that larger randomized controlled trials or systematic reviews may. It does, however, serve the purpose of keeping the field informed of new or unusual clinical presentations. In this sense, it does not represent an attempt to scientifically validate diagnostic methods, treatment techniques or technology (Zhan & Ottenbacher, 2001). The very narrow intention is to inform.

Case studies

A case study is distinct from a case report in that case studies are a type of research involving a precise, planned observation of a patient. The subject is described with detail and data is collected through observation, validated measurement instruments or other various assessment techniques. The collected data may be qualitative or quantitative data that can be used to investigate and to a small degree, prognosticate response to treatment. Case studies are considered by some to be a specific non-experimental research designs that do not manipulate or control variables. Given this case studies do not reveal causal relationships between variables. They are descriptive or exploratory in nature and allow for the examination of a hypothesis without being able to prove or disprove a hypothesis.

The exploratory nature of a case study is important. Often as observations and measurements are acquired in these studies different questions which enhance the inquiry may emerge that may not have been considered at the outset of the study. "Good" research questions are those that will enable you to achieve your aim and are capable of being answered in the research setting (Kohlbacher, 2005). The beauty of case studies is that there is an opportunity to ask questions and achieve insight in the context of the clinical interaction.

How do I do it?

The clinician should consider the following five components in preparation for executing a case study:

1 The research question(s);
2 The propositions;
3 The measurements and means for analysis;
4 Determination of how the data are linked to the propositions;
5 Criteria to interpret the findings.

Yin (1994) suggests that "how" and "why" questions are well suited for case studies. An example of an explanatory, or "how" question, for a descriptive case study may be "How does lip closure dysfunction affect bolus loss in a patient with unilateral stroke?" Or an exploratory research question may be framed as "Why does trismus occur following radiation therapy in a patient with mandibular resection?" The statement of propositions should include an intention that isn't readily understood from the question being asked. An exploratory study may state a purpose and the criteria that will be used to determine if the exploration is successful. The criteria are dependent on the measurements that are recorded and the means for analyzing the measurements. Operational definitions should be in place and well described. Furthermore, definition of the duration of the study is essential. There should be clear start and stop times or some means for describing the quantity of treatment over time to which the patient was exposed. This allows for replication of the study and encourages efforts at case comparison for clinicians consuming the study. After the data collection the question that was asked and the propositions supporting the question should be naturally linked. The data will either support the proposition or not, depending on the criteria used to interpret the findings. For a question such as "How do lip closure exercises affect bolus loss in a patient with Bell's palsy?," we could consider the following:

1 The research question:

  a How do lip closure exercises affect anterior bolus loss in a patient with unilateral stroke?

2 The propositions:

   a   The orbicularis oris and associated muscles that contribute to lip closure and bolus containment may be strengthened with specific lip-closure exercises.

3 The measurements and techniques used for analysis:

   a   The patient will be observed to take water sips in 10-ml increments for a total of 100 ml;

   b   Oral loss of liquid will be monitored for number of events;

   c   Strain-gauge measurements of isometric lip closure will be acquired before the initiation of therapy;

   d   Lip resistance exercises will be initiated daily for 30 consecutive days;

   e   At the close of 30 consecutive sessions:

      (i) The patient will be observed to take water sips in 10-ml increments for a total of 100 ml;

      (ii) Oral loss of liquid will be monitored for number of events;

      (iii) Strain-gauge measurements of isometric lip closure will be acquired.

   f   The difference in pre-treatment and post-treatment measures will be compared using descriptive statistics.

4 The proposition that strengthening the orbicularis oris and other associated muscles could be linked to increased isometric pressure measured via strain gauge measurements. Further linking of a reduction in number of events of oral loss of liquids would link the proposition that the strengthening exercises had an effect on the clinical sign.

5 The criterion for determining change = 50% reduction in oral loss events during a measurement period compared with baseline.

6 The criterion for determining resolution = 0 events of oral loss on three consecutive measurements.

Single-subject research

In contrast to the case report, single-subject research is considered to be either semi-experimental or experimental, and attempts to influence an independent variable in order to examine its effects on a dependent variable in a clinical condition. The clinician will consider the question at hand and consider the strength of the theoretical proposition.

Is there a body of evidence suggesting that the question is grounded in the existing science? During the search for evidence the clinician should consider how the questions were asked in the supporting literature. Elaboration may be necessary to construct a novel question related to existing science and to allow for a design that is explanatory. The search may also yield conventions for the appropriate units of measurement, as well as established summary statistical methods. Perhaps most importantly there should be a clinical question that motivates the effort. Ideally the clinician has experienced a clinical conundrum that is not sufficiently addressed in the available scientific literature, which affords an opening to further understand the problem at hand.

Ideally, the case to be studied is the individual who inspired the clinician to develop the proposition with the hope of solving the clinical conundrum. New patients should be selected for the investigation based on how well their history and presentation match the proposition.

In summary, the clinician is tasked to carefully develop a theoretical basis for the proposition, design a means for collecting the right data, select the right subject and then analyze the data in a coherent way. This provides an opportunity to generalize the results to other patients and create groundwork for replication and larger studies.

Single-subject research designs

Simply put, single-subject research designs (SSRD) use experimental designs that employ a single subject under both experimental conditions and as their own control. Usually there is a collection of data to characterize a baseline for function. Following this an independent variable is introduced, usually in the form of a treatment or a combination of treatment and no-treatment phases. These phases are observed and a dependent variable is measured at predetermined points in time.

If clinicians are performing this task as a clinical exercise to demonstrate the effectiveness of a treatment for the purpose of patient education or practice analysis, they may choose to graphically demonstrate the change. This allows for a simple visual inspection of the baseline and treatment phases. If a target or criterion behavior or measurement has been predetermined, the pathway to the target can be graphically inspected and explained in simple terms to a patient and family as treatment commences and can be used as an incentive to continue treatment or as a marker for concluding the treatment as the goal of the therapeutic effort is reached (Backman et al., 1997). Figure 10.1 is a graphic representation of the effectiveness of a treatment.

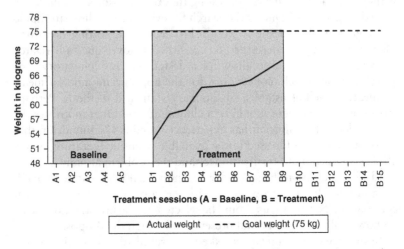

Figure 10.1 Simple goal charting. A chart graphically representing a goal
of attaining a weight of 75 kg. The clinician has recorded a
baseline weight (A1–5) and initiated therapy (B1–9), which
demonstrate progression toward the weight goal

Clinicians may also find that demonstrating a change when treatment
is withdrawn is informative. The graphic demonstration of improvement
and subsequent declination in the desired behavior may reinforce continuation of the intervention. Multiple baselines may also be enacted.
For instance, a clinician may wish to measure a baseline for duration of
mealtime and weight as dependent variables. Therapy is enacted which
is intended to increase the strength of the swallow (Figure 10.2). A theoretical proposition may be offered that greater strength will result in
less fatigue during meals. The presumption of this proposition is that
increased strength will lead to a desired and intuitive clinical measure, in
this case weight gain may be used as a dependent variable.

The purpose of this effort is to show evidence of a functional relationship between the dependent (strength and weight) and independent
(treatment) variables. Some dependent variables may covary in a positive or negative way. Ideally, the proposition suggests that the patient is
expected to gain weight while gaining strength in the propulsive components of the swallow. This would be a positive covariance. Alternately,
we may have multiple baselines and measurements in patients where there
may be a negative covariance. In Figure 10.3 scaled measurements of food
retained in the buccal cavity in a patient undergoing treatment for tongue
dysfunction go down while measurements of tongue strength go up.

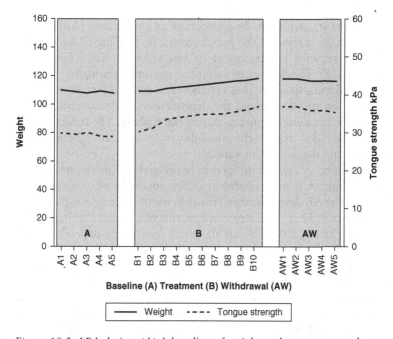

Figure 10.2 ABA design. (A) A baseline of weight and tongue strength was recorded. (B) Treatment sessions show advances in tongue strength and weight. (AW) When treatment is withdrawn a decline in both weight and tongue strength are measured

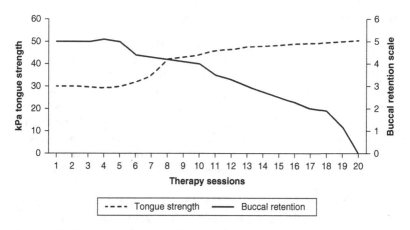

Figure 10.3 Tongue strength and buccal retention. As tongue strength increases buccal retention decreases, showing an inverse relationship between the two dependent variables

AB designs

In the simplest form these designs consist of two phases (AB). The A phase typically represents the pre-treatment or baseline phase and the B phase represents the treatment or intervention phase (Tincani & Travers, 2018). The dependent variable is measured during the A phase over several trials to assure that variation is accounted for. As treatment is applied during the B phase the dependent variable continues to be measured in the same manner as during the A phase. The collected data is then analyzed to explore the possibility of an association between the treatment and the dependent variable.

When there are striking differences between the A and B phase measures the clinician is more confident of the possibility of a relationship. However, the AB design is often criticized for not having adequate control of biases to be deemed a proper experimental design (Graham et al., 2012; Tate et al., 2013) in that the effect seen in the dependent variable could be due to some other, uncontrolled variable that is not being measured. In the natural history of stroke, patients typically rise above baseline function as they enter a post-stroke recovery phase (Cassidy & Cramer, 2017; Bernhardt et al., 2017). This spontaneous recovery often occurs without interventions and is considered an uncontrolled bias. Given this, AB designs are often considered "pre-experimental" designs in that the only measurements taken are baseline and the single treatment phases (Krasny-Pacini & Evans, 2018) pay no attention to the effect of bias. To be considered a true experimental design, it is suggested that the phase changes either be withdrawn (ABA) or repeated (ABAB).

Withdrawal (ABA) and alternating phase (ABAB) designs

To be assured of a relationship between the treatment and changes in the dependent variable a "withdrawal" design, or ABA design, is employed. Withdrawal of the intervention reintroduces the baseline condition. Ideally the ABA design demonstrates the effect of treatment when improvements or changes in the dependent variable return to levels that were witnessed in the A phase (Manolov & Onghena, 2017). This technique is particularly effective in demonstrating interventions that have an immediate effect of a direct intervention (i.e. chin tuck or head turn) on a dependent variable (i.e. clinical signs of aspiration events).

One of the problems with ABA designs is that the "withdrawal" of treatment can leave a patient in a vulnerable state because they return to an undesirable baseline that may cause further illness or discomfort, introducing ethical concerns inconsistent with good clinical care. A second problem that arises is that some treatments may have a longer-term or more permanent effect, such as training that focuses strength training. In a study involving a patient with a treatment and the expected spontaneous recovery after a stroke, a complete return to the previous baseline may not be observed after withdrawal of the treatment and a second baseline representing the stronger patient must be acquired.

Given the possibility of a differing baseline following time (i.e. stroke) or treatment (strengthening), the withdrawal approach is often considered to be a lower standard for single-case experimental design. It is recommended that at least three attempts at phase changes be enacted to move beyond the bounds of a "pre-experimental" study (Tate et al., 2013). This allows for the examination of multiple baselines as the patient progresses through the rehabilitative effort. An appropriate approach is to extend the ABA design and reintroduce the intervention phase again, creating an ABAB or alternating phase design (Figure 10.4).

Randomization

The alternating phase design can extend far beyond the baseline and three alternating phases, and may be constructed to test the treatment and withdrawal repeatedly (ABABAB) or in a randomized placement of the

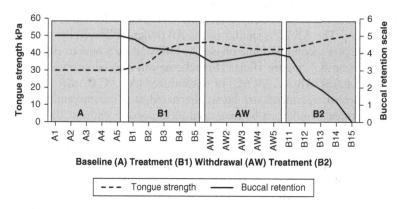

Figure 10.4 ABAB design. Therapy is withdrawn after the B phase with a difference in measurements from the initial baseline. Reintroduction of strengthening therapy after the withdrawal phase shows an increase in strength measurements and a reduction in the retention of food in the buccal cavity

A and B phases over several phases (i.e. AB BA BB AB AA BA) (Kratochwill & Levin, 2010). The randomization and alternating order make it less probable that external conditions occurring during the alternation of phases have an effect on the dependent variable being measured. Further, randomization reduces the possibility of an "order effect" which can occur when conditions are being applied in the same sequence.

Most clinically oriented, single-subject research efforts with alternating-phase designs will assume that there isn't true randomization in the phase schedule for taking measurements in the differing phases. In most clinical scenarios, obtaining baseline data assumes that the A phase will always precede any other phase in data collection and so a limited randomization of a block design is typically employed. Furthermore, the reader should not confuse the research design and order of phases during data collection with the comparisons that can be made post-data collection. For instance, a limited randomization design such as AABBABABBA can be split into different sets of comparisons, AABB–AB–AB–BA or AAB–BA–BA–BBA (Krasny-Pacini & Evans, 2018). The comparisons that are possible are now quite involved and it is imperative that measurements are taken with the same frequency and manner in each phase (Kratochwill et al., 2013).

Alternate-treatment design (ABAC)

Further variation in the withdrawal and multiple baseline designs includes the introduction of a second intervention. This is very effective for determining which of two interventions is more effective in treating a disorder. The ABAC is similar to the AB design, followed by a measurement of a second baseline phase (A) followed by a new or different intervention (C) (Figure 10.5). This scheme can also be extended over several phases (AB AC AB AC) or randomized (AB AC CA BA). When two different treatments are being alternated, it is recommended that the treatment conditions be measured in succession without the baseline (i.e. AB AC AB BC CB).

This allows for examination of both treatments and reduces the influence of one type of treatment on a succeeding treatment or the "carry-over effect" (Holcombe et al., 1994). Should carry-over be suspected a "wash-out" period, in which the individual is given more time to return to a baseline or to extinguish behaviors of a particular treatment, is suggested before introducing or after withdrawing an intervention (Skolasky, 2016).

Other considerations for multiple baseline designs

There are several advantages to multiple baseline designs. There is an improvement in internal validity as each reintroduction and withdrawal

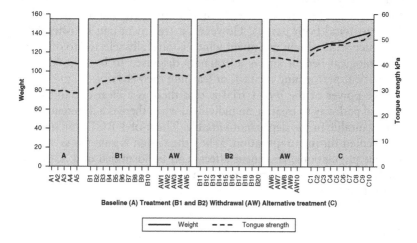

Figure 10.5 ABABAC design. A baseline (A), first treatment (B1), withdrawal (AW), followed by a second attempt at the same treatment (B2), are performed. After this another withdrawal (AW) and alternative treatment (C) are enacted

of the treatment is considered, and there are fewer opportunities for coincidental effects from unknown or unmeasured variables to affect the changes in the dependent variable (Gonnella, 1989). Another advantage of multiple baseline designs is that replication occurs within the design, allowing for a more powerful argument for the validity of the results that are observed.

Careful consideration should go into the frequency of data collection. A stable baseline should be recorded with a minimum of three data points before initiating a new phase. Five data points are preferred (Tate et al., 2013; Skolasky, 2016).

N-of-1 randomized trials

The *n*-of-1 randomized controlled trial (RCT) is a powerful single-subject research design which applies principles that are common to larger RCTs that are conventionally believed to be the standard for medical research. The *n*-of-1 RCT conducts a trial of either two differing interventions (one experimental treatment and one alternate treatment) or a single intervention and a placebo. The experimental and placebo or alternate treatments are sequenced by random assignment. In this type of design the investigator and the patient are both blinded to the treatment being offered. This is easy to achieve in pharmaceutical research where a placebo drug can be manufactured to exactly masquerade as the real drug. In behavioral and rehabilitative research it is more difficult to blind both parties. However, a treatment can be offered in sequence with a sham treatment which is carefully selected to offer no physiological benefit and is adequately disguised to be believable to the patient performing the task or learning the behavior.

The power of the *n*-of-1 trial is that there is a clear-cut and well-defined pathway to treating an individual when there is a difference that is measurable in the dependent variable. The *n*-of-1 RCTs can also be augmented through replication. When the design is run across several patient populations, treatment effects can be identified and a "meta-analysis" of the *n*-of-1 studies can be achieved (Shadish et al., 2008; Shadish, 2014).

Statistical analysis

Statistical analysis is believed to be difficult to employ in single-case designs. Repeated measures from a single individual are not considered to be independent and stability within phases is often not observed in alternating designs with multiple baselines. Recent developments in statistical manipulation allow for the fluctuation around a common mean within a phase and common residual variance within all phases, allowing for a determination of effect size between the baseline and the treatment phases (Hedges et al., 2012).

For most simple, single-subject research designs, graphic examination of the data in the form of histograms, line graphs or other means is the most apt method for communicating findings to patients and staff. Additional approaches for demonstrating change are the simple two standard deviation band method, the celeration line and the C-statistic (Zhan & Ottenbacker, 2001).

The two standard deviation band employs the calculation of standard deviation of the baseline data points with the superimposition of horizontal bands at the point of ±2 standard deviations over the graphed data (Figure 10.6). A significant effect would be achieved when at least two consecutive points acquired during the intervention phase fall outside of the band.

A celeration line is created to demonstrate where baseline data fall above or below the 50% point. During the intervention phase the data points are tracked relative to the celeration line. If there is a deviation from the baseline data, with more than 50% of the data advancing beyond the celeration line, a conclusion can be drawn that the treatment has had an effect on the dependent variable (Figure 10.7).

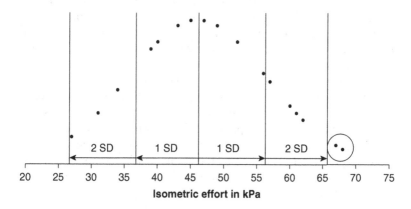

Figure 10.6 Bell curve for isometric effort. The data points are analyzed to create a bell-shaped curve with bands overlaid to represent the standard deviation from the mean. In this dataset, the two circled data points lie beyond the second standard deviation, suggesting a significant effect from treatment

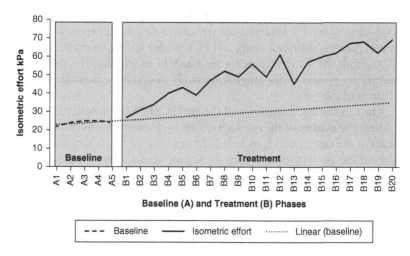

Figure 10.7 Celebration/trendline isometric effort. A baseline measurement for isometric effort is taken with treatment following. A linear trend line (the dotted linear baseline) can be generated showing the projected isometric performance without treatment. The graphic representation suggests the desired effect of treatment as the treatment data point rests above the dotted celeration line (linear baseline)

A C-statistic calculates the baseline data trend and relates this to the trend of a combination of the baseline and intervention datasets (Young, 1941). This approach only requires eight data points from the baseline and treatment phases, and provides an impression of random variation within and among the phases by reporting a *P* value. In this way the C-statistic is often used to evaluate the stability of the baseline data to determine readiness for initiation of the treatment phase. There is a risk of type 1 error due to the repeated measures of the same subject during the treatment phases. It is important to remember that the C-statistic identifies only the magnitude of the change when the treatment phase data is added to the stable baseline data. It will not allow for absolute statements with regard to whether the change was produced by the intervention (Crosbie, 1989).

Evidence

Although popular and ubiquitous, single study designs were not held in high esteem by the research community (Perdices & Tate, 2009) but this opinion changed as the designs became more sophisticated and their clinical importance was realized (Howard et al., 2015). The Oxford Centre for Evidence-Based Medicine added the *n*-of-1 RCT to the list of level 1 evidence for treatment decision purposes in individual patients (Howick et al., 2011), together with systematic reviews of multiple RCTs. Instruments to assist in examining the precision and thoroughness of the single-case study design have been developed (Tate et al., 2008).

The Single-Case Experimental Design (SCED) Scale was developed to address the quality of the research efforts by focusing on several components of the design which included the sampling of behaviors during the phases, the presentation of raw data, projected ability to replicate the findings and the potential for generalization of the findings (Tate et al., 2008). This was revised as the Risk of Bias in *n*-of-1 Trials (RoBiNT) Scale, which implemented changes in item content, scoring format, and the development of additional subscales to achieve better internal and external validity (Tate et al., 2013). Changes improving internal validity included an examination of blinding to minimize bias, with special attention given to the construction of sham treatments and surety of patient and clinician blinding. Treatment adherence is examined to assure that the planned administration of the treatment and the actual administration of the treatment were well described and documented to assure, in turn, the establishment of a functional relationship between the dependent and independent variables. Fidelity of the design is also rated with attention to independence of the person rating the patient's performance and the person delivering the treatment. External validity was purported to be improved by focusing on rating the precision of the description of the therapeutic setting, so that expectations for generalizability of the findings were confined and focused. Further detailed descriptions of the treatment were required including number, duration and periodicity of the sessions to allow for replication in a similar setting.

Conclusion

Many individuals who pursue work in clinical environments are drawn by the interactions with individual patients and their unique tribulations. The intimacy of the one-on-one struggle to achieve a positive result compels the study of single cases, whether in a randomized control or in a simple account of an unusual patient presentation. Careful construction of the effort, from the development of the proposition to the selection of measurement tools, can be refined before collecting data. The clinician is aided by reviewing and conceptually mastering the elements of the RoBiNT Scale, so that the research effort yields a clinically useful and publishable result. Most importantly each patient who comes before you hopes that his or her rehabilitative struggle is worth the labor. The single-subject endeavor establishes that you are attending to their aspirations by measuring their labor and providing a demonstration of their achievements.

References

Backman CL, Harris SR, Chisholm JAM & Monette AD. 1997, 'Single-subject research in rehabilitation: a review of studies using AB, withdrawal, multiple baseline, and alternating treatments designs,' *Archives of Physical Medicine and Rehabilitation*, 78(10), 1145–1153.

Bernhardt J, Hayward KS, Kwakkel G et al. 2017, 'Agreed definitions and a shared vision for new standards in stroke recovery research: the Stroke Recovery and Rehabilitation Roundtable taskforce,' *International Journal of Stroke*, 12(5), 444–450.

Cassidy JM & Cramer SC. 2017, 'Spontaneous and therapeutic-induced mechanisms of functional recovery after stroke,' *Translational Stroke Research*, 8(1), 33–46.

Crosbie J. 1989, 'The inappropriateness of the C statistic for assessing stability or treatment effects with single-subject data,' *Behavioral Assessment*, 11, 315–325.

Gonnella C. 1989, 'Single-subject experimental paradigm as a clinical decision tool,' *Physical Therapy*, 69(7). 601–609.

Graham JE, Karmarkar AM & Ottenbacher KJ. 2012, 'Small sample research designs for evidence-based rehabilitation: issues and methods,' *Archives of Physical Medicine and Rehabilitation*, 93(8), S111–S116.

Guyatt G, Sackett D, Adachi J et al. 1988, 'A clinician's guide for conducting randomized trials in individual patients,' *CMAJ: Canadian Medical Association Journal*, 139(6), 497.

Hedges LV, Pustejovsky JE & Shadish WR. 2012, 'A standardized mean difference effect size for single case designs', *Research Synthesis Methods*, 3(3), 224–239.

Holcome A, Wolery M & Gast DL. 1994, 'Comparative single subject research,' *Topics in Early Childhood*, 14(1), 119–145.

Howard D, Best W & Nickels L. 2015, 'Optimising the design of intervention studies: Critiques and ways forward,' *Aphasiology*, 29(5), 526–562.

Howick J, Chalmers I, Glasziou P et al. 2011, 'The 2011 Oxford CEBM evidence levels of evidence (introductory document),' Oxford: Oxford Centre for Evidence-Based Medicine, available from: https://www.cebm. net/wp-content/uploads/2014/06/CEBM-Levels-of-Evidence-2.1.pdf.

Kohlbacher F. 2005, 'The use of qualitative content analysis in case study research,' *Forum Qualitative Sozialforschung/Forum: Qualitative Social Research*, 7(1) Art. 21, available at: http://nbn-resolving.de/urn:nbn:de: 0114-fqs0601211.

Krasny-Pacini A & Evans J. 2018, 'Single-case experimental designs (SCEDs) to assess intervention effectiveness in rehabilitation: a practical guide,' *Annals of Physical and Rehabilitation Medicine*, 61(3), 164–179.

Kratochwill TR & Levin JR. 2010, 'Enhancing the scientific credibility of single-case intervention research: randomization to the rescue,' *Psychological Methods*, 15(2), 124.

Kratochwill TR, Hitchcock JH, Horner RH et al. 2013, 'Single-case intervention research design standards,' *Remedial and Special Education*, 34(1), 26–38.

Manolov R & Onghena P. 2017, Analyzing data from single-case alternating treatments designs. *Psychological Methods*, available at: http://dx.doi. org/10.1037/met0000133.

Perdices M & Tate RL. 2009, 'Single-subject designs as a tool for evidence-based clinical practice: Are they unrecognised and undervalued?', *Neuropsychological Rehabilitation*, 19(6), 904–927.

Rogers LA & Graham S. 2008, 'A meta-analysis of single subject design writing intervention research,' *Journal of Educational Psychology*, 100(4), 879.

Sackett DL. 1997, 'Evidence-based medicine,' *Seminars in Perinatology*, 21(1), 3–5.

Shadish WR. 2014, 'Analysis and meta-analysis of single-case designs: an introduction,' *Journal of School Psychology*, 52(2), 109–122.

Shadish WR, Rindskopf DM & Hedges LV. 2008, 'The state of the science in the meta-analysis of single-case experimental designs,' *Evidence-Based Communication Assessment and Intervention*, 2(3), 188–196.

Skolasky Jr RL. 2016, 'Considerations in writing about single-case experimental design studies,' *Cognitive and Behavioral Neurology*, 29(4), 169–173.

Tate RL, Mcdonald S, Perdices M, Togher L, Schultz R & Savage S. 2008, 'Rating the methodological quality of single-subject designs and *n*-of-1 trials: introducing the Single-Case Experimental Design (SCED) Scale,' *Neuropsychological Rehabilitation*, 18(4), 385–401.

Tate RL, Perdices M, Rosenkoetter U et al. 2013, 'Revision of a method quality rating scale for single-case experimental designs and *n*-of-1 trials: the 15-item Risk of Bias in *n*-of-1 Trials (RoBiNT) Scale,' *Neuropsychological Rehabilitation*, 23(5), 619–638.

Tincani M & Travers J. 2018, 'Publishing single-case research design studies that do not demonstrate experimental control,' *Remedial and Special Education*, 39(2).

Yin R. 1994, 'Discovering the future of the case study. Method in evaluation research', *Evaluation Practice*, 15(3), 283–290.

Young LC. 1941, 'On randomness in ordered sequences,' *Annals of Mathematical Statistics*, 12(3), 293–300.

Zhan S & Ottenbacher KJ. 2001, 'Single subject research designs for disability research,' *Disability and Rehabilitation*, 23(1), 1–8.

Index

Printed in the United States
by Baker & Taylor Publisher Services